Practical Clinical Epidemiology for the Veterinarian

Practical Clinical Epidemiology for the Veterinarian

Aurora Villarroel

WILEY Blackwell

This edition first published 2015 © 2015 by John Wiley & Sons, Inc

Editorial Offices

1606 Golden Aspen Drive, Suites 103 and 104, Ames, Iowa 50014-8300, USA

The Atrium, Southern Gate, Chichester, West Sussex, PO19 8SQ, UK

9600 Garsington Road, Oxford, OX4 2DQ, UK

For details of our global editorial offices, for customer services and for information about how to apply for permission to reuse the copyright material in this book please see our website at www.wiley.com/wiley-blackwell.

Library of Congress Cataloging-in-Publication Data

Villarroel, Aurora, author.
  Practical clinical epidemiology for the veterinarian / Aurora Villarroel. – First edition.
     p. ; cm.
  Includes bibliographical references and index.
  ISBN 978-1-118-47206-4 (pbk.)
  1. Veterinary epidemiology.   I. Title.
  [DNLM: 1. Epidemiologic Methods–veterinary.   2. Disease Outbreaks–veterinary.
3. Evidence-Based Practice.   SF 780.9]
  SF780.9.V55 2015
  636.089′44–dc23
                                   2014047527
A catalogue record for this book is available from the British Library.

Wiley also publishes its books in a variety of electronic formats. Some content that appears in print may not be available in electronic books.

Cover images: Vet and Cat © elenaleonova/iStockphoto

Set in 9.5/13pt Meridien by SPi Publisher Services, Pondicherry, India

Printed in Singapore by C.O.S. Printers Pte Ltd

1   2015

Dedicated to all (present and future) members of this great profession

Contents

Preface

The intention of this book is to open your eyes to the tools that epidemiology provides in the daily work of a clinician working with any animal species. This book will not help you become an epidemiologist; it is only a glimpse into what you can do with epidemiology.

So, what is epidemiology? The definition of epidemiology is the study of diseases in a population. Maybe due to the population term, most people think that epidemiology is only suited to veterinarians working with cattle or food animals in general. However, companion animal veterinarians use epidemiology every day; they do not work with individual animals in a vacuum because their patients are part of a population that interacts at the dog park, at shows, at parties, on the street, and also at the vet clinic—that is your vet clinic! We all deal with animal populations and we use epidemiological methods every day. Being aware of how to use these methods to our advantage will enable us to become better practitioners to improve the health of our patients, prevent disease, and provide the best therapeutic options.

Throughout this book, you will notice the use of the terms "disease" and "condition" interchangeably. This is because the same epidemiological methods can be used to determine the risk of a disease such as lameness or a condition such as twin pregnancies in mares, which is not a disease per se but a problem. Other "conditions" that can be studied with the same epidemiological methods are not problems but positive outcomes such as "cure," "positive response to a treatment," or "extended life," as happens with cancer treatments.

The book starts by describing the most common measurements of disease and some of the most commonly used terms in epidemiology in Chapters 1 and 2. There is a minimal part on statistics, simply to point out what are the appropriate statistical tests to be used. These tests are not explained and there are no formulas; for that you need to look into statistics books. The book continues in Chapter 3 with what I consider to be the most important part of the book: how to read and interpret research papers. Research papers are the "point of the spear" for new knowledge; however, just because something is published does not mean that it is good work, accurate, or true. My hope is that after applying the knowledge in this chapter, you will realize that you can determine whether a study warrants the conclusions that are published or not and whether you can use that information to help your patients. Chapter 4 covers in a simple straightforward manner examples of the different epidemiologic study designs to show the pros and cons, as well as the information obtained from each. Chapter 5 covers a core distinction in epidemiology: association does not mean causation. If you have ever spoken in length with an epidemiologist, you would have probably noticed that epidemiologists are very careful in the use of each term. This chapter will explain why. The final two chapters of the book will cover two of the most common uses of epidemiology encountered on the daily work at a veterinary clinic, that is, diagnostic tests (Chapter 6) and outbreak investigations (Chapter 7). In the chapter about diagnostic tests, you will learn how to evaluate the strengths and weaknesses of a test and properly interpret the results. In the chapter on outbreak investigations, you will learn how to determine the transmission pattern of a disease or condition so you can help your patients by preventing disease spread and future disease occurrence. At the end of the book, there is a section that collects all formulas in one place, as well as a glossary of the most important epidemiologic terms used throughout the book.

This book is intended to provide concise and straightforward information on how to apply epidemiological concepts in daily practice. Only the most necessary formulas and calculations will be presented, with real-life examples from all animal species, but especially focused on companion animals. Most reference articles are "open access," which means they can be downloaded for free from the Internet. My hope is that this book will help make you a better clinician.

Acknowledgments

I want to sincerely thank everyone who has made this book possible. Among them are the veterinary students who I have had the privilege to guide over the years and have taught me so much during that time. Special gratitude is due to my dear mentor Dr. V. Michael Lane, who helped me grow when I was a fledgling epidemiologist and did plant the seed for this book in my mind. He has also graciously helped me make it better with his reviews. Finally, I have to thank my family (two- and four-legged) for always allowing me to follow my dreams. Thank you all.

About the companion website

Practical Clinical Epidemiology for the Veterinarian is accompanied by a companion website:

www.wiley.com/go/villarroel/epidemiology

The website includes:

* Exercises for self-study and review

1   Describing health and disease

Disease does not occur at random; if it were we would not have a job! There is a pattern for every disease; we just need to find it.

To find how disease behaves we need to answer the following questions:
- What is the problem?
- Who gets diseased?
- Where is the disease concentrated?
- When does disease occur?

Answering all these questions (the essence of **epidemiology** is describing disease in populations) should lead us to the answer of the ultimate question we have about a certain disease (*why* does it happen?) and enable us to prevent it.

Case definition

The best explanation of the true substance of the word "definition" in matters pertinent to epidemiology comes from combining two of the meanings of the "definition": (i) an exact statement or description of the nature, scope, or meaning of something, and (ii) the degree of distinctness in outline of an object (Oxford Dictionaries online).[1] Therefore, the more carefully we describe things, the more distinctness we achieve. In defining words, it is important to avoid using another word with the same root as the one we are defining. When defining a **case**, it tends to be more complete and accurate when following the same rule of not using words with the same root.

Practical Clinical Epidemiology for the Veterinarian, First Edition. Aurora Villarroel.
© 2015 John Wiley & Sons, Inc. Published 2015 by John Wiley & Sons, Inc.
Companion website: www.wiley.com/go/villarroel/epidemiology

Example

When asked to define a diarrheic patient, simply stating it is a dog with diarrhea does not give much distinction to the case. However, if we define a diarrheic patient as a dog with feces that are not well-formed and cannot be picked up without leaving a mark on the ground gives a clear-cut characteristic that allows anyone to categorize a patient as having diarrhea or not.

What is the problem?

Before we start looking into who is diseased or where it is, we need to define what we are going to consider a diseased individual looks like; in other words, we need a **case definition**. This seems silly at first, but it is the most important step in any study or investigation and is not so clear-cut if you look deeper.

Example

Let us suppose we want to investigate if there is a problem of parvovirus in a kennel. How would you define a case of parvovirus? Most people would say a puppy with diarrhea. The problems with this simple definition of a case of parvovirus are as follows:
• There are other causes of diarrhea in puppies, so you may be overestimating how much parvovirus infection there truly is.
• Parvovirus may have asymptomatic infections, so you may be underestimating infection.
• Parvovirus can have other clinical signs without diarrhea, such as lethargy, anorexia, fever, vomiting, and severe weight loss, so you may be underestimating infection by looking only at puppies with diarrhea.
• How old can a dog be while still being considered a puppy? In other words, what is the "case definition" of a puppy?
  To get the best estimate of truly infected dogs in a population, we would have to better define a case of parvovirus infection. An example could be "dogs less than 9 months old with a positive fecal ELISA test for parvovirus." This definition would minimize the number of dogs with diarrhea due to other causes (because they have to have a positive ELISA test), and it would also minimize the number of dogs excluded because they did not have diarrhea.

The importance of case definition becomes paramount when comparing research studies about a certain disease. If two studies do not have the same case definition, the results of both studies cannot be compared directly.

Example

A study on hip dysplasia in dogs (Paster *et al.* 2005) showed that inclusion of the caudal curvilinear osteophyte in the definition of canine hip dysplasia significantly altered the diagnosis of a large proportion of dogs, usually toward a higher score but sometimes to a lower score (Figure 1.1).

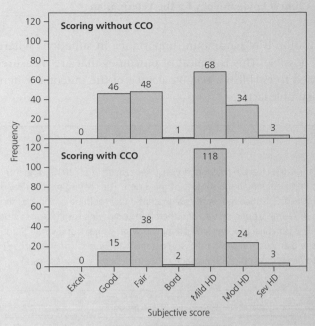

Figure 1.1 Distribution (frequency [no.]) of subjective hip scores for dysplasia using two different definitions (Paster, E.R., LaFond, E., Biery, D.N., Iriye, A., Gregor, T.P., Shofer, F.S., and Smith, G.K. (2005). Estimates of prevalence of hip dysplasia in golden retrievers and Rottweilers and the influence of bias on published prevalence figures. *Journal of the American Veterinary Medical Association*, **226**(3):387–392. © AVMA).

Another example is from a study on diagnosis of staphylococcal infections in a veterinary hospital (Geraghty *et al.* 2013). In this study, phenotypic appearance of cultured bacteria or genotypic analysis was used to determine which staphylococcal species was isolated from each animal. Figure 1.2 shows a summary of the data presented in the published paper, showing large mismatch in the results using one method versus the other.

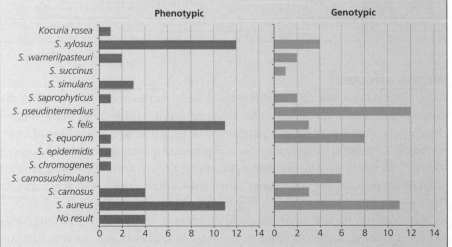

Figure 1.2 Distribution of isolation of staphylococcal species defined via phenotypic or genotypic methods (data source Geraghty, L., Booth, M., Rowan, N., and Fogarty, A. (2013). Investigations on the efficacy of routinely used phenotypic methods compared to genotypic approaches for the identification of staphylococcal species isolated from companion animals in Irish veterinary hospitals. *Irish Veterinary Journal*, **66**(1):7–15).

Case definition is of paramount importance in situations where a range of outcomes is possible. This is typical of outcomes that are measured by scores, which are used to establish a relative degree of the outcome when there is no directly measurable factor.

Example

In a study on gastric ulcers in pleasure horses (Niedzwiedz *et al.* 2013), the authors used a scoring system to determine the severity of the lesion. The scoring system they described is shown in Figure 1.3. Notice that with this description it would be possible to replicate the study using the same scoring system and therefore comparing results across studies. There could be only a potential problem in determining what "small" and what "large" lesions are—that is, a diameter threshold that would qualify a lesion as small or large. Therefore, it is better to always use objective characteristics to define cases or scores.

Lesion severity score	Description
0	No lesions
I	Lesions appear superficial (only mucosa missing)
II	Small, single, or multifocal erosions or ulcers
III	Large, single, or multifocal ulcers, or extensive erosions and sloughing
IV	Active hemorrhage or adherent blood clot

Figure 1.3 Lesion severity score description for a study on gastric lesions in pleasure horses (Niedzwiedz, A., Kubiak, K., & Nicpon, J. (2013). Endoscopic findings of the stomach in pleasure horses in Poland. *Acta Veterinaria Scandinavica*, **55**:45–55).

Who is affected?

Remember we are looking for patterns of disease, so the question is whether the entire population is affected or there are some specific **subgroups** more affected than others? Any type of subgrouping can be investigated: age, gender, breed, environment, disposition (mainly used for companionship, racing, hunting, or other), diet, etc. To continue with the parvovirus example, we know that most affected animals are puppies and young dogs. Among the young dogs it is mostly males, in theory reflecting their higher tendency to roam lose compared with females.

An example for the environmental differences can be found in feline leukemia, a disease more common in multicat households and in cats that are allowed access to the outdoors.

You can surely find an example for different diets, breeds, etc.

Where is the disease concentrated?

Defining the spatial distribution of disease may help identify risk factors and the behavior of infection. A risk factor is any characteristic that increases the risk of an animal for a certain condition. For example, which horses get infected, those in pasture or those in the barn? Is the disease spreading to adjacent stalls or are apparently "random" stalls involved? Are neighboring farms affected too? Do affected animals live in specific areas such as downtown (smog), or close to wet areas?

When does disease occur?

Is there a pattern in time? How many animals are affected in winter versus summer, spring, and fall? Is there a difference in the number of diseased individuals before and after a given event (change in disinfectant, vaccination event, etc.)? Is there a cyclical nature to the disease that could coincide with mosquito season or freezing?

Evaluate the epidemic curve–temporal distribution of cases. The first case diagnosed in an outbreak is called the "index case." A representation of the number of cases by days will show the type of epidemic curve of a disease (Figure 1.4). A "point-source" curve shows a high number of affected animals initially, which fades over time. This is typical of situations where many animals are exposed at the same time, like in outbreaks of food-borne diseases. A "propagated" epidemic curve shows a slow increase in the number of cases and a slow decrease too. This curve is typical of epidemics of infectious (contagious) diseases, where animals get exposed at different points in time (i.e., one animal gets infected and spreads the infection to a few others, which in turn infect others).

> Answering the who, what, where, and when of a disease leads to the why and how.

Types of measurements

Following are the most common ways to measure events in epidemiology, and then we will look into specific measurements of disease.

Counts

A count of individuals is used to establish the size of the population. However, when evaluating how important a disease is, simply reporting the count of sick animals does not give much useful information.

Example

If someone says they have two sick dogs, is that a little or a lot? Obviously, it depends on how many dogs they have in total. If they have two dogs, it means all of their dogs are diseased, but if it is a kennel that has 50 dogs, 2 out of 50 dogs is not a lot.

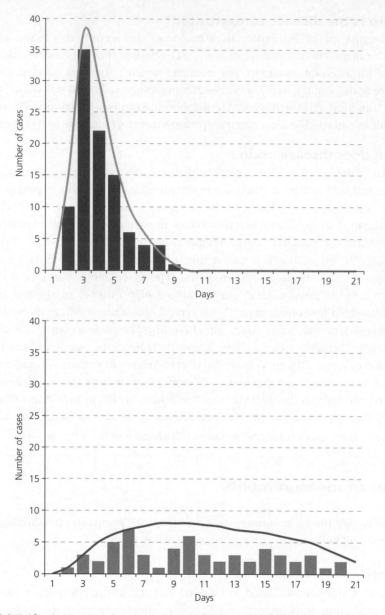

Figure 1.4 Epidemic curves: point-source (top) and propagated (bottom).

Everything has to be studied in context, in the case of epidemiology, in reference of the total population. Some may be thinking now that if we are dealing with a terrible disease that can spread very fast and kill the animals, even 2 out of 50 animals is too much. Agreed, but it is not a lot compared with 2 out of 2. We are simply looking at numbers right now; we will add meaning or significance to these numbers later in Chapter 5. The point is that, to give a sense of how big the number of diseased animals is, it needs to be put in context in reference of the size of the total population.

Proportions

A proportion is the most normal way of looking at the magnitude of the number of animals affected with a disease. It puts the count of sick animals in perspective of the number of total animals in the population.

The formula to calculate a proportion is as follows:

$$\frac{A}{A + B} \qquad\qquad (1.1)$$

where A is the number of sick animals and B is the number of healthy animals. Together A and B make the total population.

Note that the numerator is ALWAYS included in the denominator. Therefore, *proportions compare a subgroup with the whole group of animals under study*. They are usually expressed as percentages.

> **Example**
>
> Two sick dogs would represent 100% for the client that has two dogs total:
>
> $$\frac{\text{Sick}}{\text{Sick} + \text{Healthy}} = \frac{2}{2 + 0} = 1 = 100\%$$
>
> While in a kennel that has 50 dogs, they would represent only 4%:
>
> $$\frac{\text{Sick}}{\text{Sick} + \text{Healthy}} = \frac{2}{2 + 48} = 0.4 = 4\%$$

When calculating and reporting proportions, it is paramount to report what population is included in the denominator, as this may not always be clear, and simply reporting a percentage can lead to confusion as to how that proportion was calculated.

> **Example**
>
> In a study about risk factors for dystocia in Boxers (Linde Forsberg and Persson 2007), the authors show a graph (Figure 1.5) with two different proportions calculated using the same animals in the numerator but different denominator. The light bars represent the proportion of bitches within each age group (numerator) among all whelpings (denominator, $n = 253$), while the dark bars represent the proportion of bitches within each age group (numerator) among whelpings that resulted in dystocia (denominator, $n = 70$). This is not clear from the graph itself but becomes evident when reading the text.

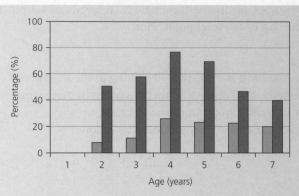

Figure 1.5 Proportion of whelpings by age group in a study on Boxers (Linde Forsberg, C. & Persson, G. (2007). A survey of dystocia in the boxer breed. *Acta Veterinaria Scandinavica*, **49**:8).

In contrast, in a study on the incidence of vaccine-induced sarcomas in cats (Dean *et al.* 2013), the authors specify that they used three different denominators to calculate the incidence of this type of tumors in their study (Figure 1.6).

Denominator   1. The total number of cats registered at the selected practices at the end of 2007.

Denominator   2. The total number of consultations/examinations, for which a code was in the system (e.g. primary consultation, repeat consultation etc.) recorded for cats by the selected practices during 2007.

Denominator   3. The total number of vaccinations visits for which there was a code in the system for vaccination visit (e.g. booster vaccination, primary vaccination courses etc.), recorded for cats by the selected practices during 2007.

Figure 1.6 Description of denominators used for the calculation of incidence of vaccine-induced sarcomas in cats (Dean, R.S., Pfeiffer, D.U., & Adams, V.J. (2013). The incidence of feline injection site sarcomas in the United Kingdom. *BMC Veterinary Research*, **9**:17–19).

Ratios

A **ratio** shows the *relationship between two mutually exclusive groups*. This means that the numerator cannot be included in the denominator. In other words, an animal cannot be part of both groups that are being compared. It is like comparing apples and oranges.

The formula to calculate a ratio is as follows:

$$\frac{A}{B}$$

(1.2)

where *A* is the number of animals in one group and *B* is the number of animals in the other group.

A typical example of a ratio you can see in the literature is the ratio of males to females. Obviously, an animal cannot be both. It is usually expressed in print with figures as *A* : *B* and with text as *A/B* or *A*-to-*B*. Verbally, it is expressed as "ratio of *A* to *B*." It does not matter which one of the two groups goes first, although there seems to be a tendency to put the lowest number last.

Example

A typical veterinary clinic may be expected to have a 5 : 1 dog-to-cat visits. This means that for each cat they see, the clinic will see five dogs. Again, it is obvious that an animal cannot be both a dog and a cat, so this is a ratio.

In another example, it has been shown that a higher adult/young ratio decreases aggression among young horses. This means that the more adult horses there are for each young horse, the better they all get along. Horses are either young or old; they cannot be both at the same time.

However, it is not always easy to determine where to draw the line to include an animal into one group or another when the characteristic that is used to classify them changes over time, as opposed to gender or breed, which are fixed. With the example of the horses, we could consider that a horse is young until 3 years of age. So a horse that is 2 years and 11 months old (35 months) will be considered "young," while a horse that is 3 years and 1 month old (37 months) will be considered old. Do we really expect much difference in behavior between these two horses? Should they be included when studying horse aggression? Should we use a different cutoff point for this study? These are some of the most common questions that arise when dealing with ratios. Notice the importance of definitions of age in this case.

Rates

A **rate** represents the speed of something developing. A rate compares a subgroup with the whole group of animals during a specific time. Therefore, it is like looking at a proportion *including the time each individual is at risk*.

The formula to calculate a rate is as follows:

$$\frac{A}{(A + B)\ \text{time}} \tag{1.3}$$

The most important feature of a rate, which makes it different from a proportion, is that it directly accounts for the time that each individual is at risk.

Example

Assume there are 2 cats staying at a boarding facility for 1 week, 3 more cats stay for 5 days, and 1 cat stays only for 2 days. Each cat has a different risk of something happening at the boarding facility because they are there for different periods of time.

   If one of them developed respiratory illness, we could say that 1 out of 6 cats or 16.7% developed disease during the time they were at the boarding facility. However, this does not give us much information because not all of the cats were exposed to the potential pathogen the same amount of time.

   To account for the different lengths of time that each cat was at risk of developing respiratory illness, we look at "cat-days," where one cat-day is any given day that a cat stayed at the boarding facility. The total number of cat-days in the example aforementioned is calculated as follows:

- 2 cats contribute 7 days each: 2 cats × 7 days = 14 cat-days
- 3 cats contribute 5 days each: 3 cats × 5 days = 15 cat-days
- 1 cat contributes 2 days: 1 cat × 2 days = 2 cat-days

Total = 31 cat-days

   Therefore, the rate of respiratory illness in this boarding facility is

$$\frac{1 \text{ sick cat}}{31 \text{ cat-days}}$$

Rates are very important when dealing with dynamic populations where animals come and go as part of the population. You are probably thinking right now that this is practically everywhere you work: your clinic, a kennel, the local shelter, a horse track, etc., and you are right. This is why epidemiology is so important to the clinical veterinarian, and why it is important to understand this measurement well. Any time when two animals are exposed unequal times to a potential risk factor for disease, we need to take those differences in "time at risk" into account.

Specific measurements of disease

There are some specific measurements of disease that are commonly used in epidemiology, giving us information about how important (quantitatively) a disease is in a given population. There are two main measurements of disease: prevalence and incidence.

Prevalence

Prevalence is a proportion that describes the number of animals that have a certain condition of interest at a given time. The formula to calculate prevalence has the number of animals that have that condition during the time of study in the numerator, divided by the number of animals at risk of developing the condition that are present at during that same time (denominator).

The formula to calculate prevalence is as follows:

$$\frac{\text{Total no. of cases}}{\text{Population at risk}} \qquad (1.4)$$

Because prevalence is a proportion, it is expressed as a percentage.

Example

Assume that in the past year you have seen 700 canine patients in your clinic, 120 of which were new puppies for their vaccinations. They all received three doses of canine distemper vaccines according to label (3–4 weeks apart before 16 weeks of age). In spite of this, 3 puppies developed signs of distemper. The prevalence of distemper among puppies in your clinic last year was 3/120 = 2.5%

Only the **population at risk** should be included in the denominator, that is, animals that can experience the event in the numerator. In the example afore-mentioned, only puppies are included, not all dogs. Other examples of accu-rately selecting the denominator for the calculation of prevalence would be including only intact males in the denominator for calculating the prevalence of testicular cancer or including only pregnant females when evaluating the prev-alence of abortions (only pregnant females can abort). This is not complicated but requires some attention.

Example A

Figure 1.7 can represent both cats at the local shelter or horses at a racetrack, whatever you prefer. Each line represents a different animal identified by name. Each column represents 1 week. The gray horizontal bars represent the presence of the animal on the premises, while each triangle represents a case of respiratory disease. Black triangles represent the first time the animal shows respiratory signs, while white triangles represent recurring cases.

The prevalence of respiratory disease during the 12-week period is as follows:
- Numerator: total cases of respiratory disease = 6 new + 2 recurring = 8 (count all triangles)
- Denominator: number of animals on the premises at any time during the period in question = 15 (count horizontal bars)

$$\text{Prevalence} = \frac{8}{15} = 0.533 = 53.3\%$$

Prevalence is expressed as a percentage; therefore, the prevalence of respiratory disease in these facilities was 53.3% during the 12-week period.

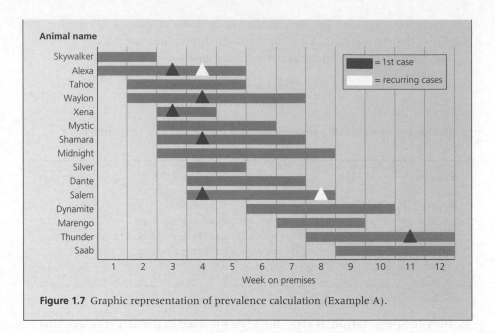

Figure 1.7 Graphic representation of prevalence calculation (Example A).

Example B

Now let us assume that we are only interested in the first 4 weeks of this period (Figure 1.8). The adjusted chart would look like this:

The prevalence of respiratory disease during this 4-week period is as follows:

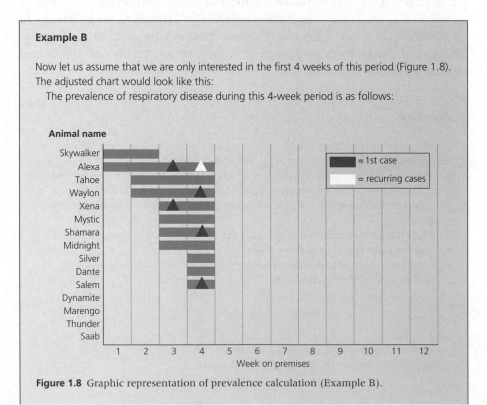

Figure 1.8 Graphic representation of prevalence calculation (Example B).

- *Numerator*: total cases of respiratory disease = 5 new + 1 recurring = 6 (count all triangles)
- *Denominator*: number of animals on the premises at any time during the period in question = 11 (count horizontal bars, not animal names!)

$$\text{Prevalence} = \frac{6}{11} = 0.545 = 54.5\%$$

Because prevalence is expressed as a percentage, the prevalence of respiratory disease in these facilities was 54.5% during the initial 4-week period.

Incidence

Incidence is a rate that describes the speed at which a given population acquires or develops a certain condition. To calculate the incidence, only the number of new cases that occurred during the evaluated period of time is included in the numerator, while the denominator takes into account the time that each animal is at risk. This is important because once an animal has acquired a certain condition (e.g., been neutered, aborted, or developed diabetes), it is not at risk of "newly" developing that condition again, at least within a certain period of time. For example, a female can abort multiple times but only when she is pregnant.

The formula to calculate incidence is as follows:

$$\text{Incidence} = \frac{\text{No. of new cases}}{\text{Population-time at risk}} \qquad (1.5)$$

Because incidence is a rate, it has to be expressed using the appropriate time units (cat-days, horse-weeks, etc.). Commonly, the reporting is done in whole integers (without decimals), although it is not compulsory. In other words, an incidence of 0.25 cases per cow-day would commonly be reported as 25 cases per 100 cow-days.

Example C

Let us go back to the example of cats in a local shelter or horses at a racetrack (Figure 1.7). The incidence of respiratory disease during the entire 12-week period is as follows:
- Numerator: only new cases of respiratory disease = 6 (count only black triangles)
- Denominator: total weeks at risk up to when an animal has its first case (count individual dark gray cells). This can be easily visualized by changing the color of the weeks once an animal has suffered a case of respiratory disease, as seen in Figure 1.9. We count only the dark gray cells (Figure 1.9).

There are a total of 48 cat-weeks or horse-weeks of exposure. Therefore, the incidence of respiratory disease in these facilities is as follows:

$$\text{Incidence} = \frac{6}{48} = 0.125$$

Expressed as 0.125 cases per cat-week (or horse-week) or as 125 cases per 1000 cat-weeks (or horse-weeks).

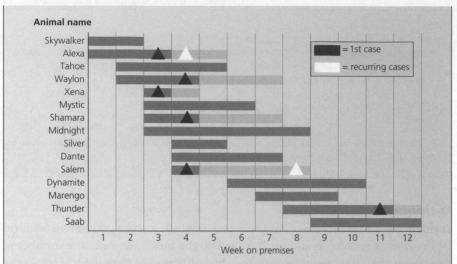

Figure 1.9 Graphic representation of incidence calculation (Example C, notice the altered colors).

Example D

If we were to look at the first 4 weeks only, the formula for calculating incidence would change to the following:
- *Numerator*: only new cases of respiratory disease = 5 (count only black triangles)
- *Denominator*: total weeks at risk up to when an animal has its first case (count individual dark gray cells) = 21

$$\text{Incidence} = \frac{5}{21} = 0.238$$

This is expressed as 0.238 cases per cat-week (or horse-week) or 238 cases per 1000 cat-weeks (or horse-weeks). The adjusted chart would look as in Figure 1.10.

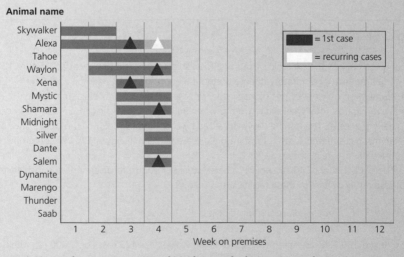

Figure 1.10 Graphic representation of incidence calculation (Example D).

Comparison of prevalence and incidence

The main differences between prevalence and incidence are as follows:

- **Prevalence** counts *all cases* in the population, while **incidence** only counts *new cases*.
- **Incidence** accounts for *differences in time* that animals are exposed to the risk of disease.

> Prevalence can be compared with a photo of an event, while incidence would be the movie.

Therefore, both the numerator and the denominator can be different when calculating prevalence and incidence in a population. The numerator will be different if there are repeated cases of disease. The denominator will include time and will be different with repeated cases of disease. The denominator would also be different in dynamic populations (varying numbers of animals at risk). Once an animal has contracted a specific condition, it may not be at risk of developing the same condition again as a "new" event, although it can be a recurrence or recrudescence of the condition. Because it cannot be considered a "new" case, it is excluded from further incidence calculations. Hopefully, the example mentioned will help understand these subtleties.

Example

In the example of cats in a shelter or horses at a racetrack, we can see that although prevalence did not change much comparing the entire 12-week period and the initial 4 weeks, incidence was almost double in the initial 4-week period compared with the entire period, which indicates that the speed of disease was faster at the beginning of the period than at the end. The movie always gives you a better idea of what is going on than a single still photo.

Because of the difference in the numerator between prevalence and incidence, it is of utmost importance to properly define a new case, with special attention to the "new" part.

Example

If the same graphs were to represent lameness cases and lameness on different legs are considered different cases, the cases represented by the white triangles could in fact now be new cases if the lameness in that animal is on a different leg (so we would represent them as black triangles for ease of visualization).

The following last few measurements of disease are not as commonly reported in the veterinary literature but are presented here for ease of reference when they are encountered.

Morbidity

Morbidity is a very specific measurement of disease defined as the proportion of animals affected with a specific condition in a given population. Thus, it is a proportion. It is a measure of the amount of disease in a population, like prevalence.

The formula to calculate morbidity is as follows:

$$\text{Morbidity} = \frac{\text{No. of cases}}{\text{Total population}} \qquad (1.6)$$

> **Example**
>
> Assume a total population of 1000 dogs (all ages) that are seen by a veterinary clinic. Assume they see 6 dogs with gastric dilation/volvulus (GDV).
>
> $$\text{Morbidity of GDV is } \frac{6}{1000} = 6\%$$

Mortality

Mortality is another specific measurement of disease defined as the number of animals that die of any cause within a population *in a specific period of time*. Thus, it is a rate and needs to include the time period in the denominator. It is also commonly referred to as crude mortality, to differentiate it from **disease-specific mortality**.

The formula to calculate mortality is as follows:

$$\text{Mortality} = \frac{\text{Total no. of deaths}}{\text{Total population-time at risk}} \qquad (1.7)$$

> **Example**
>
> Assume that from the total population of 1000 dogs seen by the veterinary clinic in the previous example, they lose 10 patients every month. For ease of calculation, we will focus on a single month.
>
> Crude mortality in the population is 10/1000 dog-months = 0.01 deaths per dog-month

Disease-specific mortality

This is another specific measurement used in epidemiology defined as the number of animals that die of a specific disease within a population *in a specific period of time*. Because it refers to mortality, it is also a rate. It is an indication as to how many animals in a population die of a specific disease. It should not be confused with case-fatality, explained next.

The formula for disease-specific mortality is as follows:

$$\text{Disease-specific mortality} = \frac{\text{No. of deaths due to the disease}}{\text{Total population-time at risk}} \quad (1.8)$$

Example

Following with the previous example, assume that 2 of the 6 cases of GDV die in spite of everything they do to help them.

GDV-specific mortality is $\dfrac{2}{1000}$ dog-months = 0.002 deaths due to GDV per dog-month

---

Case-fatality

This measurement represents the severity of a disease. It is the proportion of diseased animals (denominator) that died due to the disease (numerator).

The formula to calculate case-fatality is as follows:

$$\text{Case-fatality} = \frac{\text{No. of deaths due to the disease}}{\text{No. of cases}} \quad (1.9)$$

Example

Using the numbers from the ongoing example,

$$\text{GDV case-fatality is } \frac{2}{6} \text{ dogs with GDV} = 33\%$$

The major difference between these four measurements can be more easily understood when expressing the outcome in a full sentence:

1 GDV morbidity: 6% of dogs seen at this clinic suffer from GDV.
2 Crude mortality: 1 dog dies every 100 dog-months (for comparison with the next measurement, we can express it as 10 dogs die every 1000 dog-months).
3 GDV-specific mortality: 2 dogs die of GDV every 1000 dog-months.
4 GDV case-fatality: 33% of dogs that have GDV die.

These four measurements are more easily visualized through a Venn diagram as follows (Figure 1.11).

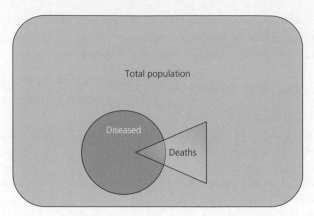

Figure 1.11 Venn diagram for the representation of specific disease measurements.

1 Morbidity would be represented as the circle divided by the rectangle.
2 Mortality: the triangle divided by the rectangle.
3 Disease-specific mortality: intersecting slice of the triangle and the circle, divided by the rectangle.
4 Case-fatality: intersecting slice of the triangle and the circle, divided by the circle.

Note

[1] http://www.oxforddictionaries.com/.

2 Basic epidemiology concepts

We will define some basic terms in this chapter to provide language for the rest of the book. Notice that some words that are commonly used in day-to-day conversations have very specific meanings in epidemiology and may imply certain things that are not common knowledge.

> **Example**
>
> When talking about a causative factor in epidemiology, it implies that a specific set of criteria have been met (Chapter 5), or otherwise we only talk about "associated" factors.

Outcome

In clinical evaluations, the **outcome of interest** is usually the presence or absence of some clinical sign, a specific disease, or nonpathologic condition such as pregnancy. The outcome of interest is the ultimate measurement that we are trying to investigate; in other words, the result or main question. Multiple outcomes can be measured in the same study.

> **Example**
>
> In a study about the effect of gold bead implantation on pain in dogs with hip dysplasia (Jaeger *et al.* 2005), the outcome was improvement of pain signs (Figure 2.1). The experimental question was "does implantation of gold beads improve pain signs in dogs with hip dysplasia?" This question begs the reporting of at least three different outcomes: improvement, no change, and worsening. Notice that the authors stratified

Practical Clinical Epidemiology for the Veterinarian, First Edition. Aurora Villarroel.
© 2015 John Wiley & Sons, Inc. Published 2015 by John Wiley & Sons, Inc.
Companion website: www.wiley.com/go/villarroel/epidemiology

even more, adding "mild" and "large" options to each end. If instead of these categories the study would have reported simply "improvement" versus "no improvement," it would have lumped in the same category those dogs that had no change and those that worsened, which would have portrayed results that could be misinterpreted as simply not changing.

Owner's guess of treatment given	Pain signs of canine hip dysplasia						
	Complete recovery	Large improvement	Mild improvement	No change in signs	Mild aggravation	Large aggravation	Total number of dogs
Placebo	0	0	1	6	2	2	11
Gold	11	28	10	3	0	0	52
Don't know	0	0	2	10	1	2	15

Figure 2.1 Changes in pain signs in dogs with hip dysplasia after treatment with gold bead implantation (Jaeger, G.T., Larsen, S., & Moe, L. (2005). Stratification, blinding and placebo effect in a randomized, double blind placebo-controlled clinical trial of gold bead implantation in dogs with hip dysplasia. *Acta Veterinaria Scandinavica*, **46**(1–2):57–68).

In a study about the effect of a specific diet (chelated form of zinc, copper, and manganese) on reproductive performance in bitches (Kuhlman and Rompala 1998), the authors measured the difference in weight change between supplemented and nonsupplemented bitches during gestation and lactation, as well as the number of puppies they give birth to (Figure 2.2). The experimental question was "what changes in dam weight over time and litter size will a specific combination of chelated minerals induce?," and therefore the outcomes were multiple.

Bitch body weight change and litter size at birth

Diet	Gestation	Lactation	Mean litter size
	kg		
Control mean (SEM; $n=17$)	3.17 (0.78)	−0.56 (0.30)	6.2[a] (0.4)
Chelated mean (SEM; $n=17$)	3.81 (0.67)	−0.95 (0.42)	7.3[b] (0.4)

[a,b] Means not sharing a common superscript letter are significantly different at $P=0.05$.

Figure 2.2 Comparison of outcomes in a study of diet effect on reproduction (Kuhlman, G. & Rompala, R.E. (1998). The influence of dietary sources of zinc, copper and manganese on canine reproductive performance and hair mineral content. *The Journal of Nutrition*, **128**: 2603S–2605S. © American Society for Nutrition).

Risk factor

Risk is defined in epidemiology as the probability of an event. A risk factor is therefore anything that can alter the probability of an event (the outcome we are investigating). This term may conjure a negative image, implying that the presence of this factor increases the risk of a negative outcome. In reality, the outcome may be positive, and then the increased **association** with the risk factor would also imply a positive property or **protective risk factor**.

Example

In the aforementioned study about the effect of mineral source on reproductive performance in bitches, chelated minerals would be considered a risk factor for larger litter size than inorganic minerals.

Comparing the risk of disease in two groups of animals that differ in only one characteristic will help identify whether that characteristic poses a risk for developing the disease. This characteristic then is called a risk factor, which is any characteristic (internal or external) that may potentially alter the "amount" or "speed" of disease in a **population at risk** of developing that disease.

Example

Being female is a major risk factor for mammary gland tumors in dogs; it does not mean that male dogs cannot develop this type of cancer, but that females have much higher rates of mammary gland tumors. This seems obvious, but can you say that the risk of prostate cancer is higher in males than in females? The answer is no because females are not at risk of prostate cancer because they do not have a prostate. Only those subgroups of the population that can be at risk of developing the disease should be compared.

To identify potential risk factors for a disease, different groups of animals need to be compared that differ only on the characteristics of that risk factor. However, in real life this is not always possible, so we match the groups as closely as possible to decrease the variation due to other characteristics.

Example

If gender is studied as a risk factor for a given disease, the incidence of this disease needs to be compared between males and females to determine if it is actually true that gender is a risk factor for that disease. All other characteristics of the animals need to be as close as possible in both males and females (e.g., age, breed, and environment).

Unit of analysis

For most studies, the unit of analysis or interest is the individual animal. However, under certain circumstances, the unit of analysis could be a group of animals (higher-level aggregate) such as a cattery, a kennel, or a barn, while in other situations the unit of analysis could be a part of an animal (lower level) such as each eye, each ear, or each leg.

Examples

In a study of the effect of partnering with the community to improve live releases in animal shelters in the USA (Weiss *et al.* 2013), all animals (dogs and cats) that were taken in by a specific shelter had shared characteristics because of the idiosyncrasies of that shelter (e.g., more volunteers, closer to town, and better funding). Therefore, the unit of analysis was the shelter (Figure 2.3) and not the individual animals.

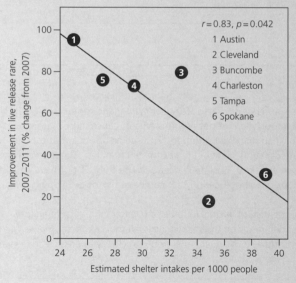

Figure 2.3 Effect of number of intakes on improvement in live-release rate in US animal shelters (Weiss, E., Patronek, G., Slater, M., Garrison, L., & Medicus, K. (2013). Community partnering as a tool for improving live release rate in animal shelters in the United States. *Journal of Applied Animal Welfare Science*, **16**(3):221–238).

Another example comes from a study of the epidemiology of parasites in horse farms in three European countries (Samson-Himmelstjerna *et al.* 2009). Because all horses in a barn were exposed to the same environment and management, the unit of analysis becomes the facility and not the individual horses. Additionally, the authors of this study determined that facility type (FT; riding stable, stud, or racehorse stable) had similar characteristics that allowed using FT as the unit for certain analysis such as the one shown in Figure 2.4.

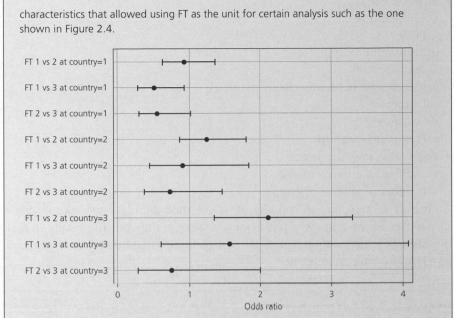

Odds ratios with 95% Wald confidence limits for strongyle infections risk between farm types (FT, i.e. l=riding stable, 2=stud farm, 3=racehorse stable) for the three countries involved (i.e. l=Germany, 2=Italy, 3=UK).

Figure 2.4 Comparison of risk of strongyle infection in three facility types and across three European countries (Samson-Himmelstjerna, G., Traversa, D., Demeler, J., Rohn, K., Milillo, P., Schurmann, S., Lia, R., Perrucci, S., di Regalbono, A.F., Beraldo, P., Barnes, H., Cobb, R., & Boeckh, A. (2009). Effects of worm control practices examined by a combined faecal egg count and questionnaire survey on horse farms in Germany, Italy and the UK. *Parasites & Vectors*, **2**(Suppl. 2):S3).

Variables

A **variable** is any identifying characteristic that can have different values (including yes/no) or different "versions."

Examples of variables
- *Gender*: Male or female
- *Breed*: Appaloosa, Arabian, Paint, Thoroughbred, etc.
- *Age*: Weeks, months, or years
- *Reproductive status*: Intact or castrated/spayed/neutered
- *Hair coat*: Long versus short, colors, wired versus soft hair, etc.

In our daily work as veterinarians, we collect multiple measurements about our patients. These are all variables that we collect to provide information so we can make decisions but that does not mean they are all outcome variables. Typical examples of variables measured in daily clinical practice are as follows:

- Physical exam
  - Temperature
  - Pulse
  - Respiration
- Diagnostic tests
  - Blood work (CBC and chemistry panel)
  - Urinalysis
  - Cultures
  - Pregnancy diagnosis
- Population measurements
  - Number of animals exposed
  - Number of animals affected

It may be tempting to consider all of the measurements we take during a physical exam or diagnostic test as outcomes or results but the reality is that, depending on the question that is being asked, these variables may be an outcome or a risk factor for an outcome.

Example

We can compare the average temperature of horses that have a culture positive for *Salmonella* versus those that have a negative culture. In this case, temperature is the outcome variable, while the culture result is an exposure or risk factor.

If instead we ask how many horses with fever have a positive culture for *Salmonella*, then the outcome variable is the proportion of cultures that are positive, while temperature is a potential risk factor that can be evaluated in the analysis.

Example 1 (Saarto *et al.* 2010)

Background: The aim of the study was to investigate the effect of acupuncture on wound healing after soft tissue or orthopaedic surgery in dogs.

Methods: 29 dogs were submitted to soft tissue and/or orthopaedic surgeries. Five dogs had two surgical wounds each, so there were totally 34 wounds in the study. All owners received instructions for post operative care as well as antibiotic and pain treatment. The dogs were randomly assigned to treatment or control groups. Treated dogs received one dry needle acupuncture treatment right after surgery and the control group received no such treatment. A veterinary surgeon that was blinded to the treatment, evaluated the wounds at three and seven days after surgery in regard to oedema (scale 0–3), scabs (yes/no), exudate (yes/no), hematoma (yes/no), dermatitis (yes/no), and aspect of the wound (dry/humid).

Results: There was no significant difference between the treatment and control groups in the variables evaluated three and seven days after surgery. However, oedema reduced significantly in the group treated with acupuncture at seven days compared to three days after surgery, possibly due the fact that there was more oedema in the treatment group at day three (although this difference was nor significant between groups).

Conclusions: The use of a single acupuncture treatment right after surgery in dogs did not appear to have any beneficial effects in surgical wound healing.

Figure 2.5 Abstract of a study on the effect of acupuncture on wound healing in dogs (Saarto, E.E., Hielm-Bjorkman, A.K., Hette, K., Kuusela, E.K., Brandao, C.V., & Luna, S.P. (2010). Effect of a single acupuncture treatment on surgical wound healing in dogs: a randomized, single blinded, controlled pilot study. *Acta Veterinaria Scandinavica*, **52**:57).

The outcome variable was wound healing defined in terms of aspect of the wound (dry/humid); edema score; and presence of scabs, exudate, hematoma, or dermatitis (Figure 2.5). So the study question was "does the use of acupuncture one single time after surgery (exposure or risk factor) accelerate wound healing in dogs?"

Example 2 (Vos and Ducharme 2008)

The purpose of this paper was to identify factors that would positively or negatively affect the short-term survival rate of foals with septic arthritis. Medical records of 81 foals (≤ seven months of age) with a clinical diagnosis of septic arthritis, referred to the equine hospital at Cornell University Hospital for Animals, between 1994 and 2003 were reviewed. Signalment, age at presentation, number of affected joints, joint fluid parameters, bacterial agents, treatment modalities and year of treatment were compared between survivors and non-survivors. Sixty-two of 81 foals (77%) were discharged from the hospital and classified as "survivors." Multiple joint involvement and detection of intra-articular Gram-negative, mixed bacterial infection and degenerate neutrophils were negatively associated with short-term survival. Initiation of treatment within 24hrs of onset of clinical signs and combination of treatment modalities were positively correlated with survival. Further investigation is needed to determine if these two factors have a similar influence on athletic performance.

Figure 2.6 Summary of a study on survival in foals with septic arthritis (Vos, N.J. & Ducharme, N.G. (2008). Analysis of factors influencing prognosis in foals with septic arthritis. *Irish Veterinary Journal*, **61**(2):102–106).

The outcome variable was short-term survival in foals that were diagnosed with septic arthritis (Figure 2.6). The exposure variables studied were various, of which multiple joint involvement and detection of intra-articular Gram negative, mixed bacterial infection and degenerate neutrophils were determined to be negative risk factors, while early onset of treatment and combination of treatment modalities were considered helpful for survival (protective).

Example 3 (Mellgren and Bergvall 2008)

Abstract

Background: A retrospective study of rabbits treated against cheyletiellosis was performed to evaluate the efficacy and safety of selamectin or ivermectin in clinical practice.

Methods: Medical records from 53 rabbits with microscopically confirmed *Cheyletiella* infestation were collected from two small animal clinics. The rabbits were divided into three groups, based on treatment protocols. Group 1 included 11 rabbits treated with ivermectin injections at 200–476 µg kg^{-1} subcutaneously 2–3 times, with a mean interval of 11 days. In Group 2, 27 rabbits were treated with a combination of subcutaneous ivermectin injections (range 618–2185 µg kg^{-1}) and oral ivermectin (range 616–2732 µg kg^{-1}) administered by the owners, 3–6 times at 10 days interval. The last group (Group 3) included 15 rabbits treated with selamectin spot-on applications of 6.2–20.0 mg kg^{-1}, 1–3 times with an interval of 2–4 weeks. Follow-up time was 4 months–4.5 years.

Results: Rabbits in remission were 9/11 (81.8%), 14/27 (51.9%) and 12/15 (80.8%) in groups 1, 2 and 3, respectively.

Conclusion: All treatment protocols seemed to be sufficiently effective and safe for practice use. Though very high doses were used in Group 2 (ivermectin injections followed by oral administration), the protocol seemed less efficacious compared to ivermectin injections (Group 1) and selamectin spot on (Group 3), respectively, although not statistically significant. Controlled prospective studies including larger groups are needed to further evaluate efficacy of the treatment protocols.

Figure 2.7 Summary of a study about treatment regimen options against *Cheyletiella* infestation in rabbits (Mellgren, M. & Bergvall, K. (2008). Treatment of rabbit cheyletiellosis with selamectin or ivermectin: a retrospective case study. *Acta Veterinaria Scandinavica*, **50**:1–50).

> The outcome variable was remission of *Cheyletiella* infestation in rabbits (Figure 2.7).
> The exposure variable was treatment with either selamectin or two different regimen using
> ivermectin. The study question detailed in the published paper was "how effective and
> safe are selamectin and ivermectin for the treatment of cheyletiellosis in rabbits?" Given
> that the authors compared three different treatment regimens, the effective study question
> became "which one of the three treatment regimens was better to resolve *Cheyletiella*
> infestation in rabbits?" or possibly "are all three treatment regimens similar in resolving
> *Cheyletiella* infestation in rabbits?"

Types of variables

According to their relationship to each other, there are two main types of
variables:

- **Dependent variables** are the outcomes of study as they depend on the risk
  factors.
- **Independent variables** are the risk factors, which is why they are also called
  input variables.

   For statistical purposes, variables are classified into two groups as follows:

- **Continuous variables** are those with an objective (measureable) interval
  between values, which is always the same between adjacent values. These are
  the variables that are typically measured with some kind of instrument or
  counted. They are also called **parametric variables**.

   For example, in the measurement of temperature, the difference between 98
and 99°F is 1°F, which is exactly the same difference between 104 and 105°F.
Other examples include pulse, respiratory rate, electrolyte and hormone
concentration in a chemistry panel, or neutrophil count in a CBC.

- **Categorical variables** are those with a subjective value, where the intervals between adjacent values cannot be objectively measured. They are also
  called **nonparametric variables**. These are the variables that typically
  classify animals into groups with different names and are therefore also
  called **nominal variables**. Some variables are divided in groups that indicate
  some kind of order, such as "slight," "medium," and "heavy" or using numerical
  scores such as body condition score (BCS) from 1 to 5; in this case, they are
  called **ordinal variables**. It is impossible to determine if the difference between "slight" and "medium" is the same as the difference between
  "medium" and "heavy." This is also called discrimination of variables. The
  use of numerical scores can confuse people into thinking that those
  are continuous variables, but asking the question of whether the difference
  between a pain score 1 and a score 2 is the same as the difference between
  a pain score 3 and a score 4 will show that this is a noncontinuous variable,
  that is, a categorical variable.

   Examples of categorical variables are gender (intact male, intact female,
spayed, or neutered), breed, BCS, pain score, and any variable that can be

classified with words such as "yes/no"; "slight, medium, and heavy"; or "some, moderate, and excessive."

> Continuous variables are objectively measured and categorical variables are subjectively scored.

Any continuous variable can be translated into a categorical variable, by setting up cutoff limits for inclusion into one of the categories or the other. However, categorical variables cannot be transformed into continuous variables. Because of this, it is always advisable to collect and record objective data. There is always time to transform the data into different categorical variables later.

Examples

When age is measured in years, it is a continuous variable (a year is a year, no matter if it is the difference between 1 and 2 years of age or 8 and 9 years of age). Age can be translated into a variable that only has two categories: young and old, where young is considered to be any animal up to 3 years of age and old is defined as age after that point. Clinicians may set the break point between these categories at different ages (2, 3, 4, or even 5 years). Most clinicians may elect to divide this variable into three categories: young, medium-aged, and old. When age data is recorded only as young, medium-aged, or old, it will never be possible to know the actual age in years.

Another example is temperature; when measured with a thermometer, it will be a specific number of degrees (Fahrenheit or Celsius), and therefore it is a continuous variable (a degree is a degree). However, fever is a categorical variable that can only have values of "yes" or "no." For a dog, fever is present when the rectal temperature is above 102.5°F (39°C), while for a horse the break point is at 101.5°F (38.5°C). When data is recorded on the physical exam as presence or absence of fever, it will never be possible to know exactly how high the fever was.

Appropriate statistical analyses for continuous/parametric variables

Continuous variables are compared using the mean and the **standard deviation** (SD). The mean gives an average value of the variable for all animals measured in the group. The SD is a measure of the spread of the data in that group; the larger the SD, the larger the range of values.

Example

Let us compare the mean heart rate and the SD for the following two groups of cats:

Group A
Cat 1: 155 bpm
Cat 2: 170 bpm

Cat 3: 185 bpm
Cat 4: 230 bpm
Mean = 185 bpm, SD = 32.4

Group B
Cat 5: 180 bpm
Cat 6: 185 bpm
Cat 7: 185 bpm
Cat 8: 190 bpm
Mean = 185 bpm, SD = 4.1
Although both groups have the same mean heart rate, group A has a wider range of values than group B, as indicated by the larger SD.

SD versus standard error of the mean

It is common to confuse these two measures because they are reported in the literature in a very similar way (mean ± SD and mean ± standard error (SE)), but each one has its specific meaning:
- SD describes the actual variability of a measurement among animals in a group.
- SE indicates the **precision** of measurement of the mean if we were to take different samples in a population.

Example

Assume we have 10 horses in a barn and we calculate the mean temperature of those horses. The SD is a measure of the variation of temperature we found in that barn (i.e., if the range was wide or not). The **standard error of the mean** (SEM) will tell us how precise this measurement of the mean is. If we were to use this mean to represent the average temperature of all horses in the world, the SEM gives us a range within which we have a certain level of confidence that true mean for all horses would lie within.

The SD is a measure of variability within a group of animals (individual-level data). The SEM is an indication of how certain we are that the mean measured in our group is reflective of the mean in similar animals in other places (mean-level data).

We will not go deeper into analyses for continuous variables as that falls into the realm of statistics. Suffice it to list the most common methods to be used for comparison of continuous variables between groups of animals:
- Student's T-test to compare means between two groups.
- ANOVA to compare means between three or more groups.
- Paired T-test to compare means in the same group of animals measured twice (such as before and after an intervention); for pairs of animals (such as twins); or for pairs of structures within an animal (such as left and right eye).
- Correlation coefficient measures the change in a continuous variable as a function of the change in another continuous variable (both variables implicated are continuous).

- Linear regression evaluates the effect of one or more risk factors on a continuous outcome variable, assuming the relationship is linear. When more than one risk factor is included in the equation, it becomes a multivariate regression.

Appropriate statistical analyses for categorical/nonparametric variables

Categorical variables should be compared using counts and percentages of animals included in each category. When ordinal numerical scores are used, it is possible to compare the median, which indicates the ordinal value below which 50% of the measured animals are, while the other 50% would be above that value. However, it is not an easy statistic to interpret, which is why it is not recommended to use numerical scores to categorize variables. Researchers are tempted to use a parametric statistic to analyze variables that have numerical values, while they feel more confident comparing percentages of animals within a category when the categories are described with words such as "emaciated," "thin," "normal," "heavy," and "obese" as opposed to 1, 2, 3, 4, and 5.

Example

Assume a group of five dogs with BCS of 2, 2, 3, 4, and 4. The median score is 3. This seems simple because the median and the mean are equal. Now assume a group of five other dogs with BCS of 3, 3, 3, 3, and 5. The median score is also 3. However, the interpretation in both groups is confusing: half of the dogs have a BCS of 3 or less, and half have a BCS of 3 or more. In the first group it is intuitive, but in the second group it is confusing.

   However, if we were to say in the first group 20% (1/5) of dogs had BCS = 3 while in the second group it was 80% (4/5) of dogs, it is easier to compare the two groups of dogs.

   As before, we will not go deeper into analyses for categorical variables but leave that for statistics books. Here is the list of the most common methods to be used for comparison of categorical variables between groups of animals:

- Z test to compare proportions of animals in two groups.
- Chi-square test to determine if proportions of animals in two groups are different than expected.
- Fisher's exact test to determine if proportions of animals in two groups are different than expected, when any of the groups has fewer than five animals.
- Mann–Whitney U test to compare medians in two groups.
- Wilcoxon signed-rank test to compare medians in the same group measured twice.
- Logistic regression evaluates the effect of multiple risk factors on a categorical outcome variable.

- Survival analysis (Kaplan–Meier plot) evaluates the time elapsed between exposure and outcome. The outcome does not need to be death as implied by the name "survival analysis" (Figure 2.8). In fact, the outcome does not even have to be considered a "failure" but can be something positive such as hospital discharge or healing (Figure 2.9).

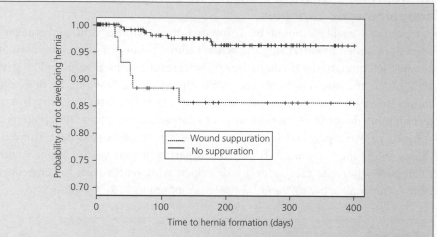

Figure 2.8 Example of the use of survival analysis to compare time to a negative event that is not "death." In this example, the event is hernia formation after colic surgery in horses that had wound suppuration or not (French, N.P., Smith, J., Edwards, G.B., & Proudman, C.J. (2002). Equine surgical colic: risk factors for postoperative complications. *Equine Veterinary Journal*, **34**(5):444–449. © Wiley).

The use of appropriate and inappropriate statistical analyses in the veterinary literature has been subject of multiple papers published in different veterinary journals. These papers tend to explain the issues in a way that is easier to understand for clinicians compared with many statistics and epidemiology textbooks (Figure 2.10).

Appropriate statistical analyses for multiple samples taken from the same animal

When studies require taking multiple samples of the same animal over time to evaluate changes, they violate one of the cardinal rules (assumptions) necessary for most statistical analyses: independence between measurements. These are called repeated measures studies, and they require specific statistical analyses that take into account the fact that different measurements in the same animal are not independent of each other. It is a common mistake to sample a few animals several times and in the analyses assume that each sample represents a different animal, when in fact they do not. Here is where it becomes crucial to identify what is the unit of analysis: it is the animal or the sample?

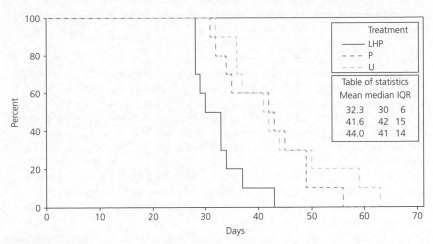

Figure 2.9 Example of the use of survival analysis to compare time to a positive event. In this example, the event is wound healing after 3 different treatment options: LHP©, cream (1% hydrogen peroxide); P, petrolatum; or U, untreated (Toth, T., Brostrom, H., Baverud, V., Emanuelson, U., Bagge, E., Karlsson, T., & Bergvall, K. (2011). Evaluation of LHP(R) (1% hydrogen peroxide) cream versus petrolatum and untreated controls in open wounds in healthy horses: a randomized, blinded control study. *Acta Veterinaria Scandinavica*, **53**:45–53).

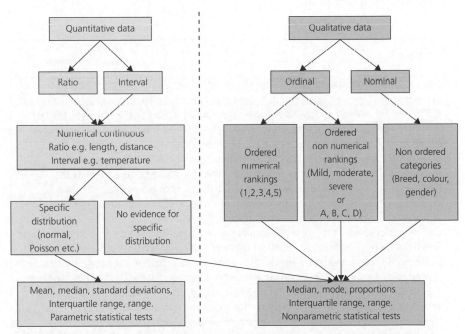

Figure 2.10 Graphic representation of the decision flow for determining the appropriate statistical comparison of common veterinary studied variables (Boden, L. (2011). Clinical studies utilising ordinal data: pitfalls in the analysis and interpretation of clinical grading systems. *Equine Veterinary Journal*, **43**(4):383–387. © Wiley).

Example

Assume a study that samples six elephants, monthly, over a period of 6 months. That makes a total of $6 \times 6 = 36$ samples, which sounds a lot better than six samples. However, the six samples belonging to each elephant are not equivalent to one sample taken from six different elephants. Consider the implications if one of the six elephants had liver disease (unknown to the researcher) and the samples are taken to evaluate the effect of a specific diet on glucose concentration in serum; now six samples would have skewed results because they all are from the same elephant with liver disease.

There are intrinsic characteristics within each individual that make those six samples related to each other. In other words, the maximum variability between multiple samples taken from the same animal can never be as much as the maximum variability between samples from two different animals.

One situation in which multiple measurements can be taken on the same animals and analyzed with statistical tests that only apply to independent measurements is when the multiple measurements performed on one animal are combined to produce a single measurement or outcome point. This method is commonly used to reduce the error of measurements and therefore increase the reliability of each data point.

Example

In a study on tylosin-responsive diarrhea in dogs (Kilpinen *et al.* 2011), the authors instructed the owners to perform daily fecal scores (1 to 5—hard to watery, at 0.5 increments), and for analysis purposes the authors averaged the scores of the last 3 days of the 7-day treatment regimen (Figure 2.11). Notice that this study shows one of the most common mistakes in analysis of scores as recently discussed, where categorical data (scores) are analyzed as continuous variables. It is impossible to establish whether the difference between a score of 4.5 and 5 is the same as that between a score of 2.5 and 3. Two appropriate methods of analyzing these data would have been (i) using the median score of those last 3 days of treatment, although this would likely show nonsignificant differences due to potential small differences in some scores, and (ii) calculating the proportion of time that the score was below a certain threshold. This last method allows for certain flexibility such as including the entire treatment regimen instead of simply the last 3 days. A dog that started with a score of 4.5 (diarrhea) and evolved throughout the days as 4.5, 4, 4, 3, 2.5, and 3 would be recorded as 50% (3/6) of days with a score below 4. We do not take into account the score on the day that treatment was initiated (7 days of treatment, 6 days of evaluation). An alternative analysis would be to obtain only one data point per dog, represented by the fecal score of the day after the last treatment dose.

Abstract

Background: The macrolid antibiotic tylosin has been widely used to treat canine chronic diarrhea, although its efficacy is based on anecdotal reports and experimental studies in dogs and not on strong scientific evidence. The term tylosin-responsive diarrhea (TRD) refers to diarrheal disorders responding to tylosin therapy within a few days. In TRD, the stool remains normal as long as tylosin treatment continues, but diarrhea reappears in many dogs within weeks after discontinuation. The aim of our trial was to assess the effect of tylosin on fecal consistency compared with a placebo treatment in dogs with suspected TRD and additionally to establish whether tylosin in dogs with recurrent diarrhea is as effective as empirical studies and anecdotal reports suggest.

Methods: Subjects comprised 71 client-owned dogs that, according to the owners, had previously been treated successfully with tylosin due to recurrent diarrhea of unknown etiology. At the initial examination, where there were no signs of diarrhea, the dogs were randomly assigned in a 2:1 ratio to a tylosin or placebo group. During a two-month follow-up the owners evaluated the fecal consistency according to previously published guidelines. When diarrhea recurred, either tylosin (25 mg/kg q 24 h, 7 days) or placebo treatment was initiated orally. Treatment outcome was evaluated as the mean of fecal consistency scores assigned during the last three days of the treatment period. To test for differences between the tylosin and placebo group in the proportion of responders, Pearson's Chi-squared test and Fisher's exact test were applied.

Results: Sixty-one dogs met the selection criteria and were followed for two months. During the follow-up 27 dogs developed diarrhea and either tylosin or placebo treatment was started. The proportion of dogs with normal fecal consistency at the end of treatment was 85% (17/20) in the tylosin group and 29% (2/7) in the placebo group (Pearson's Chi-squared test $p = 0.0049$ and Fisher's exact test two-sided, $p = 0.0114$).

Conclusions: Our findings indicate that tylosin is effective in treating recurrent diarrhea in dogs. The dose of 25 mg/kg once daily appears sufficient. No changes specific to TRD were detected in the examinations.

Figure 2.11 Abstract of a study on tylosin-responsive diarrhea in dogs (Kilpinen, S., Spillmann, T., Syrja, P., Skrzypczak, T., Louhelainen, M., & Westermarck, E. (2011). Effect of tylosin on dogs with suspected tylosin-responsive diarrhea: a placebo-controlled, randomized, double-blinded, prospective clinical trial. *Acta Veterinaria Scandinavica*, **53**:26).

It becomes obvious that there can be multiple ways of evaluating the outcome(s) of a study, but it is important to remember that only if the appropriate study design is applied and the appropriate statistical tests are used, will the results be meaningful.

Control groups

Assume the prevalence of *Bordetella* spp. infection in a kennel is 10%. Is this a problem? In other words, is this high, low, or average? The answer to this question will not be known until the prevalence in this kennel is compared with the prevalence in other kennels. Therefore, there is *always the need for a baseline comparison group* commonly referred to as the **control group**.

- **Positive control** group is a group of animals exposed to a factor that we know has an effect on the outcome, so we can tell that the exposure is in fact effective.
- **Negative control** group is a group of animals that are either not exposed at all or are exposed to a factor that will not have an effect on the outcome (**placebo** or sugar pill).

Example

Consider a mastitis study in cows to compare two treatments (A and B), where each of the four quarters of the udder will be part of a different **study group** (Figure 2.12):
- Front left—not inoculated, not treated (negative control)
- Front right—inoculated, not treated (positive control)
- Rear right—inoculated, treatment A
- Rear left—inoculated, treatment B

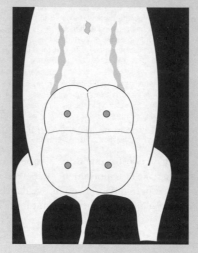

Figure 2.12 Diagram of the udder of a dairy cow (ventral view).

Sample size and *P*-value

After identifying the outcome(s), the risk factors, and how many study groups will be compared, it is necessary to calculate how many animals will be required in each group to ensure that the results are reliable. The reliability of the results will be determined by statistical analyses and the resulting probability value or **P-value**. The interpretation of the *P*-value is the probability that the results obtained in the study may be due to chance alone. A small *P*-value indicates that the probability of the outcome and the risk factor to appear associated in that way due to chance alone is small, and therefore a true association is much more likely.

Studies with large sample sizes will have more reliable results than studies with small sample sizes. Studies with large sample sizes achieve smaller *P*-values. When a study is being designed, it is important to calculate the **sample size** needed to determine if the results are reliable or not. We are not going to go into detail into how to calculate the sample size; there are free calculators online and in smartphone apps that do all the legwork. However, it is important to know

Example

For example, in Figure 2.13, extracted from a study of postoperative complications in horses recovering from colic surgery (French *et al.* 2002), let us look at the effect of wound suppuration on incisional herniation (highlighted line). The *P*-value of 0.9% (*P*=0.009) means that if we were to do the same study 1000 times, we would obtain the same association (**odds ratio** (OR) = 4.32) only nine times if this were a random event (i.e., if the result were due to chance alone). This means that because it is such a rare probability of this result to happen randomly, a true association between the risk factor (wound suppuration) and the outcome (herniation) likely exists.

Variable	Coef. (ß)	SE	OR/HR*	95% CI	P value
Jugular thrombosis					
PCV (per unit)	0.068	0.030	1.07	1.01, 1.14	0.022
Heart rate >60 beats/min	0.916	0.461	2.50	1.10, 6.17	0.044
Postoperative ileus					
PCV (per unit)	0.063	0.028	1.07	1.01, 1.13	0.021
Pedunculated lipoma	1.161	0.438	3.19	1.35, 7.53	0.010
Re-laparotomy					
EFE (y/n)	1.439	0.550	4.23	1.43, 12.39	0.016
Ileus (y/n)	1.357	0.481	3.88	1.51, 9.97	0.008
Incisional herniation—Cox proportional hazards model					
Wound suppuration (y/n)	1.464	0.557	4.32	1.45, 12.9	0.009
Heart rate (beats/min)	0.036	0.012	1.04	1.01, 1.06	0.002
Postoperative colic—Cox proportional hazards model					
LCT >360 (y/n)	1.14	0.302	3.13	1.73, 5.65	<0.001
Re-laparotomy (y/n)	1.22	0.304	3.39	1.87, 6.15	<0.001

*Hazard ratio (HR) reported for variables in Cox proportional hazards models. y/n = yes/no.

Figure 2.13 Risk factors for postoperative complications in 311 horses recovering from colic surgery. EFE, epiploic foramen entrapment; LCT, large colon torsion; PCV, packed cell volume (French, N.P., Smith, J., Edwards, G.B., & Proudman, C.J. (2002). Equine surgical colic: risk factors for postoperative complications. *Equine Veterinary Journal*, **34**(5):444–449. © Wiley).

that a calculator will require the baseline level of the outcome of interest (measurement in the control group) and the magnitude of the difference between the study group and the control group that you want to be able to detect (hint: select a value that is biologically significant to you). Then the sample size calculator will determine the number of animals required in each group to prove that this difference is true and not due to chance alone. Sample size in the results is commonly expressed as *N* or *n*.

Error and bias

Error and **bias** are characteristics that interfere with the reliability of a study. They are based on the ability of the study to conclude correctly what is the reality of the situation.

Error refers to the reliability or precision of the study. There are two types of error:

- **Type I error**—concluding that study groups are different when in reality they are not. When studying the effect of a treatment, a type I error occurs when the conclusion is that the studied treatment has an effect when in reality it does not.
- **Type II error**—concluding that study groups do not differ when in reality they are different. When studying the effect of a treatment, a type II error occurs when the conclusion is that the treatment has no effect when in reality it does.

This may be easier to understand in a 2×2 table (Table 2.1).

Table 2.1 Graphic representation of the types of errors in statistical analyses.

		Reality	
		Study groups <u>are</u> different, the treatment has an effect	Study groups are NOT different, the treatment has no effect
Decision based on the study	Study concludes that study groups <u>are</u> different, the treatment had an effect	Correct decision Power	Type I error α
	Study concludes that study groups are NOT different, the treatment had no effect	Type II error β	Correct decision

The shaded cells provide the correct interpretation, the white cells provide the errors.

Example

Assume a hypothetical study of the effect of feeding sweet potato on diabetes in dogs. If the study concludes that feeding sweet potato is associated with an increase of diabetes and this is true, then it would always happen in the overall dog population in the entire world (external validity). This is what we look for in studies to estimate the reality of the situation.

If for whatever reason, this result were not true (feeding sweet potato did not increase diabetes), then there would have been a type I error in the study because the conclusion was that there was an effect of treatment (feeding sweet potato) on the outcome (diabetes) when in reality there is not one.

On the other hand, if the conclusion were that feeding sweet potato had no effect on diabetes and in reality this effect existed, then there would have been a type II error in the study.

These types of errors are accounted for in statistical analyses as follows:

- α is the probability of making a type I error (concluding that the treatments are different when in reality they are not).
- β is the probability of making a type II error (concluding that the treatments do not differ when in reality they do)
- **Power** is the probability of correctly identifying differing treatments (concluding that the treatments are different when the treatments do in fact differ), in other words, the probability of not making a type II error. Power is equal to $1 - \beta$.

Commonly, the threshold value to accept that the results are likely not due to chance are set at $\alpha = 0.05$ (P-value of 5%) and $\beta = 0.80$ (80%). This means that we accept a 5% probability that the result of the study happened due to chance alone. In other words, if we were to repeat the same study 100 times and the treatments were in fact not different, we would get the same result only five times (due to chance).

These thresholds can be changed in situations where there are tight budget constraints or there is a biological limitation such as with diseases that have very low prevalence. Setting $\alpha = 0.05$ means that we would like to have a P-value of 5% for our results. The results are then presented with a specific resulting P-value (e.g., $P = 0.031$ or $P = 0.387$) or simply as $P \leq 0.05$ or $P > 0.05$ meaning that the results are above or below the set threshold (α). You have probably seen this multiple times in the veterinary literature. A P-value smaller than the target α means that (up to that probability) the result is likely not due to chance alone and can be considered real. A P-value larger than α means that there is a larger probability that the result can occur by chance alone.

Confidence interval

In research articles, the resulting measurements of disease or association of risk factors are frequently presented with a range of numbers in parentheses that indicate the 95% **confidence interval** (CI) of the value in front of the parenthesis. This range of values indicates how confident we can be, based on the sample size that was used, that the strength of association (value in front of the parenthesis) is indeed as it resulted. It indicates the variability of the result if the study were performed multiple times. The wider the range, the less confident we can be. The 95% CI corresponds to a P-value of 5%. If the study were performed allowing a probability of committing a type I error of 10% ($\alpha = 0.10$), then the appropriate CI to be presented in the results would be the 90% CI. This is somewhat complicated to explain in abstract, but it will make sense in the following example.

Examples

In the data presented earlier about horse colic postoperative complications, the authors reported the 95% CI of the OR for several conditions (Figure 2.13). The 95% CI for "hernia formation" when there was wound suppuration shows that the OR of 4.32 could in fact be anywhere between 1.43 and 12.39. In other words, if this same study were repeated 100 times, 95 times the OR would lie between 1.43 and 12.39, while the remaining five times it would have a value out of that range (either above or below). The biological interpretation of this range is that hernia formation can be anywhere from a slight change (OR = 1.43) to 12 times as much (OR = 12.39) that found in horses that did not have wound suppuration.

Let us now look at "heart rate" as a factor for hernia formation; it shows an OR of 1.04, with a 95% CI between 1.01 and 1.06. This means that if we were to repeat the study 100 times, we would find an OR between 1.04 and 1.06 in 95 of those experiments, while in five occasions it would be out of the range. So, we can be fairly confident that each additional heart beat per minute (at admission) was associated with a 4–6% increased probability (95% CI 1.04–1.06) of hernia formation. For additional examples and clarification of the interpretation of the OR, please refer to Section "Odds ratio".

In a study of wild boar parasite burden, the authors show two different levels of significance in a single table (Fernandez-de-Mera *et al.* 2003). For prevalence of parasitism, they show 95% CI, while for the intensity of parasitism within each animal they show 90% CI (Figure 2.14).

Another example (Figure 2.15) ties together the sample size, *P*-value, and CI. This study is a meta-analysis that compares results from several studies on the same subject, in this case, the association of serum alkaline phosphatase and survival in dogs with appendicular cancer (Boerman *et al.* 2012). Notice that cited studies with small sample size (Tham *n* = 21, Selvarajah *n* = 32) have the widest 95% CI. The lines in the graph represent the width of the CIs, while the squares represent the nominal value of the hazard ratio (also called OR, see Section "Odds ratio").

	Imported				
	n	Prevalence		Intensity	
		%	CI (95%)	Mean	CI (90%)
G. urosubulatus	9	11.1	0–48	3.00	0.00–0.00
O. dentatum	9	22.2	3–60	23.50	3.00–23.50
Metastrongylus sp.	9	66.7	30–92	633.0	21.17–1245
A. suum	9	44.4	14–79	3.00	1.00–4.75
G. pulchrum	9	0.0	0–34	NA	0
A. strongylina	9	11.1	0–48	1.00	0.00–0.00
P. sexalatus	9	22.2	3–60	1.50	1.00–1.50
S. paradoxa	9	22.2	3–60	1.50	1.00–1.50
T. suis	9	33.3	7–70	117.67	6.00–214
C. garfiai	9	11.1	0–48	1.00	0.00–0.00
M. hirundinaceus	9	0.0	0–34	NA	0

Figure 2.14 Sample size (*n*), prevalence (% and 95% CI), and intensity of parasitation (average and 90% CI) among wild boars in Spain. CI, confidence interval (Fernandez-de-Mera, I.G., Gortazar, C., Vicente, J., Hofle, U., & Fierro, Y. (2003). Wild boar helminths: risks in animal translocations. *Veterinary Parasitology*, **115**(4):335–341. © Elsevier).

Meta analysis

Study name	Sample size	Hazard ratio	Lower limit	Upper limit	Z-Value	p-Value	Hazard ratio and 95% CI	Relative weight
				Statistics for each study				Relative weight
Saam 2010(uva)	63	0.900	0.437	1.854	-0.286	0.775		11.12
Selvarajah 2009(uva)	32	2.439	1.094	5.438	2.179	0.029		9.62
Philips 2009(mva)	138	2.270	1.437	3.586	3.513	0.000		18.68
Tham 2008(uva)	21	1.660	0.481	5.728	0.802	0.423		4.82
Kow 2008(uva)	67	2.160	1.003	4.651	1.968	0.049		10.25
Kirpensteijn 2002(uva)	99	1.802	1.003	3.238	1.970	0.049		14.47
Garzotto 2000(uva)	61	1.240	1.057	1.455	2.639	0.038		31.03
		1.620	1.208	2.173	3.222	0.001		

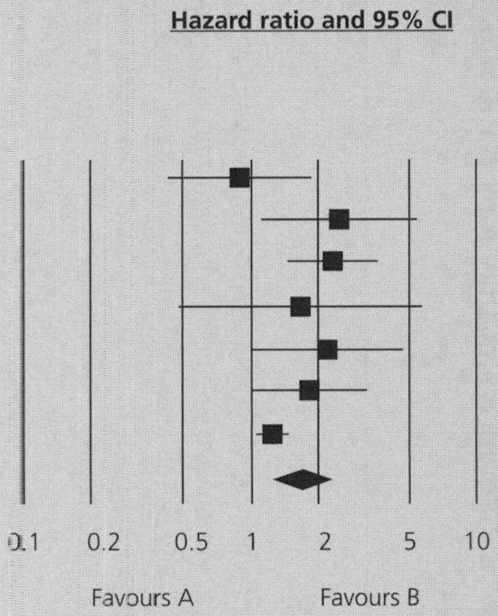

0.1 0.2 0.5 1 2 5 10

Favours A   Favours B

Figure 2.15 Meta-analysis of the association of serum alkaline phosphatase and survival time in dogs with appendicular cancer (Boerman, I., Selvarajah, G.T., Nielen, M., & Kirpensteijn, J. (2012). Prognostic factors in canine appendicular osteosarcoma—a meta-analysis. *BMC Veterinary Research*, **8**:56–58).

Bias

There is a special type of error that receives a descriptive name; it is the systematic error or bias. Bias occurs when there is a tendency to a specific outcome that is not due to the true nature of the situation (hence systematic). Commonly, bias is due to some risk factor not being accounted for in the analyses, but sometimes it happens subconsciously when the person measuring the outcome of interest knows which animals received each treatment and they are partial or "perceive" a difference and they look harder for small signs that validate their perception.

Example

Assume a study looks at the healing effect of a new topical zinc product on wounds in horses using a scoring system from 0 to 5; 0 being complete healing (i.e., no damage) and 5 being no healing at all. If the barn manager of one of the study locations had not told the researchers that the diet of all horses in that barn included a special mineral supplement that has good levels of zinc, the results of the study could be biased, because both control and treatment horses in that barn would probably heal better than other horses elsewhere because of the supplemented zinc. This would bias the results. Assume that in another study, the same person who applies the product is the person scoring the outcome; then it is possible that she/he wants the product to work so well that horses that are not healing well (score=4) are scored as moderately healing (score=3).

To avoid the bias due to subjective interpretation or perception, it is common to "blind a study," which means that the person(s) evaluating the outcome cannot administer the treatment. You may have heard of "double-blind" studies, which are common in human research, where both the subject receiving the treatment and the evaluator are blinded to whether the patient is in the control or the treatment group.

To avoid the bias due to not accounting for some risk factors in the study, it is common to standardize the characteristics of the study individuals during the selection process (e.g., breed and age) and to collect as much information as possible from the patients so that this information can be compared in all of them to determine if they are different before starting the study. This information is commonly presented in the first table of a study report, as descriptive statistics of the study.

There are several special types of bias, which are as follows:

• **Selection bias**—typical of studies where animals are selected haphazardly, such as selecting the first 10 dogs that come through the door. It is possible that those dogs that come to the clinic first thing in the morning are owned by people who are very concerned about their beloved dog and they may be giving extra supplements and extra care that make those dogs not representative of the normal dog population.

- **Detection bias**—typical of nonblinded studies, where the investigator "really" wants to find something in the treatment group and subconsciously spends more time examining animals in one group than in the other.
- **Recall bias**—typical of surveys, where it is more likely for people to remember things that happened recently or that had a significant impact on their lives, while other things are easily overlooked.
- **Information bias**—also typical of surveys, especially those with open-ended questions, where some people are more likely to give short answers and others like to give extensive answers. The amount of information collected from both would not be comparable.

Example

In a study on the effect of gold bead implantation on pain in dogs suffering hip dysplasia (Jaeger *et al.* 2005), after a period in which the study was blinded to the dog owners and data on pain perception by the owners were recorded while they did not know whether their dog had been implanted or received the placebo, owners were allowed to choose gold bead implantation for their animals. At this point, all owners knew whether their dogs had the implant or not, and the results were compared with those obtained during the blinded part of the study (Figure 2.16).

Treatment	Pain signs of canine hip dysplasia						Total number of dogs
	Complete recovery	Large improvement	Mild improvement	No change in signs	Mild aggravation	Large aggravation	
Blinded gold	5	17	8	6	0	0	36
Open gold	1	14	9	2	4	2	32

Figure 2.16 Comparison of pain perception changes after gold bead implantation during a blinded study and when owners were not blinded (Jaeger, G.T., Larsen, S., & Moe, L. (2005). Stratification, blinding and placebo effect in a randomized, double blind placebo-controlled clinical trial of gold bead implantation in dogs with hip dysplasia. *Acta Veterinaria Scandinavica*, **46**(1–2):57–68).

Confounding

Confounding occurs when another variable is "confusing" or distorting the effect that a risk factor has on an outcome. There are several characteristics that a variable needs to meet to be considered a confounding variable, which are as follows:
- It needs to be a risk factor for the outcome.
- It needs to be associated with the risk factor under study.
- It cannot be in the causal pathway between the risk factor under study and the outcome.

Example

Assume a study looking at the effect of school-trip visits (risk factor) on the cortisol levels (outcome) as an indicator of stress in tigers kept at a zoo. On school-visit days (both risk factors are associated), zookeepers let the lions out into the enclosure adjacent to the tigers, which requires the activation of the electric fence that makes a buzzing sound that makes the tigers nervous (i.e., the electric fence is a risk factor for high cortisol levels in the tigers). The electric fence is not in the causal pathway of the children making the tigers nervous; in other words, it is not a necessary part of the connection between the children and the nervousness of the tigers. The electric fence used for the lions would be a confounder of the effect that a group of screaming children would have by itself on the cortisol levels of the tigers.

Taking into account these characteristics, it can be argued that most studies are subject to confounding, especially to variables we do not know about yet. However, there are techniques to minimize the possibility of confounding through proper study designs (Chapter 4).

Interaction

Interaction occurs when two risk factors that are associated with the outcome are present at the same time and the resulting effect is modified from exposure to only one of the risk factors. This is why some people use the term "effect modification" to refer to interaction. In statistical analyses, most often this will be represented by a multivariate model that shows the effect modifying one variable will have on the outcome while maintaining all other variables unchanged. Sometimes, published studies will include interaction terms into a model showing the specific effect that a combination of variables has on the outcome. This will become clearer with some examples.

Example

In a study of rabies vaccination efficacy in dogs, vaccination success (defined as titers above the Office International des Epizooties (OIE) standard) was affected, among other variables, by breed size and number of vaccinations. This can be gleaned from the very small P-value that both variables have in the univariate analysis table (Figure 2.17), which looks at each risk factor by itself (hence the name UNIvariate—meaning analyzing one variable at a time). Their combined effect is later confirmed in the multivariate model (Figure 2.18), which analyzes multiple variables at once. In the multivariate analysis it can be seen that, using very small–small breeds with one vaccination as the reference category to which all others are compared with, rabies vaccination success was 2.25 times higher (OR = 2.25) in large breed dogs vaccinated once (highlighted) but 2.44 times smaller (OR = 0.41, transformed as 1/0.41 = 2.44 for interpretation; see Section "Odds ratio" for more information) in small breed dogs vaccinated twice (highlighted). Therefore, rabies vaccination success varied by whether dogs had one or two injections (within the same breed size). It also means that rabies vaccination success varied by breed size among dogs that had one single injection and among those that had two injections.

Variable	Level	Number of animals	Proportion of dogs with antibody titres ≥ 0.5 IU/ml, %	P-value in the univariable logistic regression analysis
Type of vaccine	1:Vaccine A	3571	87.4	
	2:Vaccine B	3218	96.9	<0.001
Day of antibody testing after last vaccination	1: 120 - 150 days	5156	92.6	
	2: 151 - 180 days	1613	90.3	0.003
Number of vaccinations	1: Once	1766	85.7	
	2: Twice	5023	94.1	< 0.001
Age at vaccination	1: < 6 month	1635	89.5	
	2: 6-11.9 months	1050	92.6	
	3: 1-2.49 years	1692	93.8	
	4: 2.5 - 4.99 years	1053	92.6	
	5: ≥ 5 years	698	90.4	< 0.001
Breed size	1: Very small/small pure-breed (< 30 cm in height)	1482	94.1	
	2: Small/medium sized pure-breed (30-45 cm in height)	1203	92.2	
	3: Medium/large pure-breed (46-60 cm in height)	1965	91.4	
	4: Large/very large pure-breed (> 60 cm in height)	1345	88.4	
	5: Unknown size mixed breeds	747	94.5	< 0.001
Gender	1: Bitch	3637	91.4	
	2: Dog	3152	92.5	0.12

Figure 2.17 Univariate analysis of the effect of different factors on the efficacy of rabies vaccination in dogs (Berndtsson, L.T., Nyman, A.K., Rivera, E., & Klingeborn, B. (2011). Factors associated with the success of rabies vaccination of dogs in Sweden. *Acta Veterinaria Scandinavica*, **53**:22).

Variable	β	SE(β)	OR[a]	95% CI[b] (OR[a])	P-value
Intercept	−1.44	0.19	—	—	—
Vaccine					
A: Nobivac	Ref	—	—	—	—
B: Rabisin	−1.47	0.12	0.23	0.18, 0.29	< 0.001
Interactions					
Breed size × no of vaccinations					
Very small -small breed size × vaccinated once	Ref	—	—	—	—
Small - medium breed size × vaccinated once	0.07	0.27	1.07	0.63, 1.84	0.79
Medium - large breed size × vaccinated once	0.68	0.21	1.97	1.29, 3.00	0.002
Large - very large breed size × vaccinated once	0.81	0.22	2.25	1.45, 3.49	< 0.001
Unknown size (mixed breed) × vaccinated once	−0.41	0.38	0.66	0.32, 1.39	0.28
Very small -small breed size × vaccinated twice	−0.90	0.24	0.41	0.25, 0.65	< 0.001
Small - medium breed size × vaccinated twice	−0.31	0.22	0.73	0.47, 1.13	0.16
Medium - large breed size × vaccinated twice	−0.61	0.21	0.54	0.36, 0.82	0.004
Large - very large breed size × vaccinated twice	−0.07	0.21	0.93	0.62, 1.42	0.75
Unknown size (mixed breed) × vaccinated twice	−0.91	0.29	0.40	0.23, 0.72	0.002
Age at vaccination × number of day after **vaccination a.b. titres were tested**					
<6 month × day 120−150	Ref	—	—	—	—
6−11.9 month × day 120−150	−0.40	0.17	0.67	0.48, 0.93	0.018
1−2.49 years × day 120−150	−0.67	0.16	0.51	0.38, 0.70	< 0.001
2.5−4.99 years × day 120−150	−0.63	0.18	0.53	0.38, 0.75	< 0.001
≥5 years × day 120−150	−0.41	0.19	0.66	0.45, 0.96	0.032
<6 month × day 151−180	−0.10	0.20	0.90	0.60, 1.35	0.62
6−11.9 month × day 151−180	−0.24	0.25	0.78	0.48, 1.29	0.34
1−2.49 years × day 151−180	−0.63	0.22	0.53	0.34, 0.82	0.004
≥2.56 years × day 151−180	−0.12	0.24	0.89	0.56, 1.42	0.62
≥5 years × day 151−180	0.58	0.25	1.80	1.10, 2.93	0.019

[a]OR = odds ratio.
[b]CI = confidence interval.

Figure 2.18 Multivariate analysis of the effect of different factors on the efficacy of rabies vaccination in dogs (Berndtsson, L.T., Nyman, A.K., Rivera, E., & Klingeborn, B. (2011). Factors associated with the success of rabies vaccination of dogs in Sweden. *Acta Veterinaria Scandinavica*, **53**:22).

3 Evidence-based medicine for the veterinarian

Evidence-based medicine (EBM) has become a buzz word in recent years to the point that it almost evokes malpractice if you do not use it or refer to it. In essence, EBM promotes the use of scientific evidence when making medical decisions, adapting new information and technology as it becomes available to improve outcomes. However, EBM does not imply to forget about personal experience as another piece of information to ultimately provide the best care possible to the patient at hand, given each particular background and circumstances.

Thoughtful practitioners plan on practicing EBM. The distinctive problem comes from "what is considered as 'evidence'?" In the distant past, given the limited spread of new knowledge to the practitioner, there was little access to new information. Therefore, most practitioners relied on their accumulated experience and that of their close peers as "evidence." Nowadays, with the immediate access to information, the problem is almost the opposite; there is so much information available that it is difficult to determine what is acceptable as evidence and what is not.

EBM focuses on "scientific" evidence. So the distinctive feature becomes "what can be considered 'scientific'?" The answer is, unfortunately, that not everything that is published is scientific evidence. A lot of the information available nowadays is nothing more than personal opinion of someone who has had the time and inclination to write it down and post it somewhere on the Internet or in a magazine. This is referred to as "gray literature." Other types of publications included in the gray literature are government publications, conference proceedings, masters and doctoral theses, newsletters, and do not forget Wikipedia, where anyone can edit an entry and write their opinion without the need of review. However, the lack of need of review does not mean that nobody can review something if she/he wants to. In this sense, Wikipedia is becoming more accurate over time, when

Practical Clinical Epidemiology for the Veterinarian, First Edition. Aurora Villarroel.
© 2015 John Wiley & Sons, Inc. Published 2015 by John Wiley & Sons, Inc.
Companion website: www.wiley.com/go/villarroel/epidemiology

multiple reviewers actually exercise their ability to edit, but there is no controlled or systematic process to the review. This systematic review process is the distinctive feature of "peer-reviewed" articles found in scientific journals. However, not all articles in a scientific journal are peer-reviewed.

In general, there are four types of articles that are commonly found in scientific journals:

- **Review articles**: They cover a disease or condition in as much depth and breadth as is known at that time using information from previously published papers (Figure 3.1). Therefore, review articles should include a large number of references to original studies or case reports that can prove the validity of a specific statement. There is usually no new information in a review article, but all available information up to that point should be included, making this type of article a good starting point when dealing with a new disease or condition. Review articles do not commonly use statistical analyses but are peer-reviewed.

- **Original studies**: They cover a specific question within a disease or condition (Figure 3.2) and therefore will include references to previous studies that show how the authors reached the study question and those studies that investigate a similar or closely related question, so they can evaluate their results in perspective with current knowledge. Most original studies require the use of statistical analyses to determine whether their results are statistically significant or due to chance alone. These are the bulk of the research papers, and their intention is to show new information. Original articles are usually peer-reviewed.

- **Case reports**: They describe new diseases or conditions in one animal or a small group of animals (Figure 3.3), in which statistical analyses are not possible. References are limited to specific points that can help the reader interpret the analogy with other diseases or a similar disease in another animal species. Case reports are usually peer-reviewed.

- **Editorials**, **Opinion**, and **White papers**: In these papers, authors express their opinion about a disease (Figure 3.4), condition, or situation, and they are the most commonly used route to express consensus reached in panel meetings (Figure 3.5). These papers tend to not use many references or statistical analyses and are not usually peer-reviewed as they pertain specifically to authors' opinions.

Examples

In a *review article* on epilepsy in cats (Pakozdy *et al.* 2014) as shown in Figure 3.1, there is a specific statement that refers to "…an established staging system for feline temporal lobe epilepsy based on the observation on a kindling model.25" The *original study* that reported the establishment of this staging system (no. 25 in that article) is a study published 40 years earlier (Wada *et al.* 1974), which is presented in Figure 3.2.

Epilepsy in Cats: Theory and Practice

A. Pakozdy, P. Halasz, and A. Klang

The veterinary literature on epilepsy in cats is less extensive than that for dogs. The present review summarizes the most important human definitions related to epilepsy and discusses the difficulties in applying them in daily veterinary practice. Epileptic seizures can have a wide range of clinical signs and are not necessarily typical in all cases. Whether a seizure event is epileptic can only be suspected based on clinical, laboratory, and neuroimaging findings as electroencephalography diagnostic techniques have not yet been developed to a sufficiently accurate level in veterinary medicine. In addition, the present review aims to describe other diagnoses and nonepileptic conditions that might be mistaken for epileptic seizures. Seizures associated with hippocampal lesions are described and discussed extensively, as they seem to be a special entity only recognized in the past few years. Furthermore, we focus on clinical work-up and on treatment that can be recommended based on the literature and summarize the limited data available relating to the outcome. Critical commentary is provided as most studies are based on very weak evidence.

Key words: Diagnosis; Etiology; Review; Seizure; Terminology; Therapy.

Figure 3.1 Summary of a review paper (Pakozdy, A., Halasz, P., & Klang, A. (2014). Epilepsy in cats: theory and practice. *Journal of Veterinary Internal Medicine*, **28**(2): 255–263. © Wiley).

Epilepsia, 15:465-478, 1974
© Raven Press, New York

Persistent Seizure Susceptibility and Recurrent Spontaneous Seizures in Kindled Cats

Juhn A. Wada, Mitsumoto Sato, and Michael E. Corcoran

Summary

Daily unilateral electrical stimulation of initially subconvulsive amygdala resulted in progressive development of seizures (kindling) in cats, culminating in generalized convulsive seizures of focal onset that could occur spontaneously. Kindled cerebral epileptogenicity persisted for up to 12 months and was characterized by (1) interictal spike discharges of consistent morphology and localization, and (2) an "all or none" response to stimulation at the generalized seizure triggering threshold. Pentylenetetrazol (Metrazol) enhanced the frequency of interictal discharge without changing its localization or morphology, and caused generalized seizures with focal onset exactly like those produced by unilateral stimulation of the amygdala. These findings indicate that repeated electrical stimulation of amygdala produces widespread alteration of brain function resulting in a permanent state of epileptogenicity. Kindling thus qualifies as an experimental model reminiscent of certain types of human epilepsy.

Figure 3.2 Summary of an original study (Wada, J.A., Sato, M., & Corcoran, M.E. (1974). Persistent seizure susceptibility and recurrent spontaneous seizures in kindled cats. *Epilepsia*, **15**:465–478. © Wiley).

This is a good place to point out that when referencing an idea or a particular finding, the original study should always be used no matter how old it is. Credit should be given where credit is due: the original researchers that had the idea, studied a new condition, or published a new finding. The best way to think of it is as always giving the credit for inventing the light bulb to Thomas Edison instead to Dr. X, who recently decided to use light bulbs in an interesting way. Dr. X will get credit for the new interesting use of the light bulb, but Thomas Edison gets the credit for inventing the light bulb.

The same aforementioned review article (Pakozdy *et al.* 2014) presents a table summarizing possible adverse effects of therapeutic products used for epilepsy in cats (Figure 3.6). All the findings shown in this table are product of multiple studies that need to be referenced (right column). Some of these studies are *original studies* that conducted an experiment to evaluate an outcome, but others are *case reports* such as reference number 61 (Ducote *et al.* 1999), which reported that phenobarbital could show skin eruptions as a possible adverse effect, from the report of hypersensitivity to phenobarbital in a single cat (Figure 3.3).

CASE REPORT
Suspected hypersensitivity to phenobarbital in a cat

J M Ducote*, J R Coates, C W Dewey, R A Kennis

Adverse reactions to phenobarbital administration have been reported in humans and dogs. This case history describes a young domestic shorthair cat that presented with clinical signs compatible with an adverse drug reaction to phenobarbital. Clinical signs included depression, anorexia, cutaneous eruptions, and a severe, generalised lymphadenopathy. These signs began approximately 21 days after beginning phenobarbital administration. Similarities between this reaction and the anticonvulsant hypersensitivity syndrome are demonstrated and possible aetiologies are discussed.

Figure 3.3 Summary of a case report paper (Ducote, J.M., Coates, J.R., Dewey, C.W., & Kennis, R.A. (1999). Suspected hypersensitivity to phenobarbital in a cat. *Journal of Feline Medicine and Surgery*, 1:123–126).

EQUINE VETERINARY JOURNAL
Equine vet. J. (1977), 9 (4), 183-185

The Legal Responsibilities of the Veterinary Surgeon arising from Advances in Equine Cardiology and in the Prescription of Drugs for Racehorses

E. CAZALET
Temple, London

SUMMARY

The paper examines the responsibilities of the veterinary surgeon in relation to the advances more recently made in the field of equine cardiology. Notwithstanding such advances it is stated that the normal established legal principles apply, in particular in relation to the preparation of certificates, namely that the veterinary surgeon must be sufficiently expert to give the opinion sought, that he must make himself fully aware of the purpose for which the certificate is required and that he must make clear the nature and limitations of any examination carried out.

The paper also refers to the current problem relating to the use of drugs in racehorses and emphasises that when a veterinary surgeon is prescribing any such drug for therapeutic purposes he must clearly warn the trainer of the danger of the drug proving positive on a laboratory test. If possible he should be in a position to state the safe period required to enable the horse to eliminate the drug from its system.

Figure 3.4 Summary of an opinion paper (Cazalet, E. (1977). The legal responsibilities of the veterinary surgeon arising from advances in equine cardiology and in the prescription of drugs for racehorses. *Equine Veterinary Journal*, 9:183–185. © Wiley).

Exploration of developmental approaches to companion animal antimicrobials: providing for the unmet therapeutic needs of dogs and cats

AAVPT Workshop White Paper Committee

Committee Members:

M. APLEY*

R. CLAXTON**

C. DAVIS[+]

I. DeVEAU[++1]

J. DONECKER[+]

A. LUCAS[††]

A. NEAL[++2] &

M. PAPICH[+++]

*Kansas State University; **Schafer Veterinary Consultants; [+]University of Illinois; [++1]U.S. Pharmacopeia, Inc. (currently with U.S. FDA); [+]Pfizer, Inc.; [††]Elanco Animal Health; [++2]U.S. Pharmacopeia, Inc. (currently with U.S. FDA-CVM); [+++]North Carolina State University

AAVPT Workshop White Paper Committee. Exploration of developmental approaches to companion animal antimicrobials: providing for the unmet therapeutic needs of dogs and cats. J. vet. Pharmacol. Therap. 33, 196–201.

The American Academy of Veterinary Pharmacology and Therapeutics (AAVPT) and the United States Pharmacopeia (USP) co-sponsored a workshop to explore approaches for developing companion animal antimicrobials. This workshop was developed in response to the shortage of antimicrobials labeled for dogs and cats, as there is a shortage of approved antimicrobials for the range of infectious diseases commonly treated in small animal practice. The objective of the workshop was to identify alternative approaches to data development to support new indications consistent with the unmet therapeutic needs of dogs and cats. The indications for currently approved antimicrobials do not reflect the broader range of infectious diseases that are commonly diagnosed and treated by the veterinarian. Therefore, the labels for these approved antimicrobials provide limited information to the veterinarian for appropriate therapeutic decision-making beyond the few indications listed. Industry, veterinary practice, and regulatory challenges to the development of new antimicrobial indications were discussed. The workshop resulted in short- and long-term recommendations. Short-term recommendations focus on the use of additional data considerations for product labeling. Long-term recommendations center on legislative or regulatory legal initiatives. The workshop recommendations will need collaboration from industry, academia, and regulatory authorities and a legal shift in the drug approval and availability processes.

Figure 3.5 Summary of a white paper (Apley, M., Claxton, R., Davis, C., DeVeau, I., Donecker, J., Lucas, A., Neal, A., & Papich, M. (2010). Exploration of developmental approaches to companion animal antimicrobials: providing for the unmet therapeutic needs of dogs and cats. *Journal of Veterinary Pharmacology and Therapeutics*, **33**(2): 196–201. © Wiley).

Oral antiepileptic treatment for cats.

Medicine	Dosage	Possible Adverse Effects	Notes
Phenobarbital	1–5 mg/kg q12h	Sedation, ataxia, PU/PD/PP, leukopenia, thrombocytopenia, lymphadenopathia, skin eruptions, coagulopathia	Serum level monitoring (100–300 µmol/L, 23–30 µg/mL)
Diazepam	0.2–2 mg/kg q8–24h	Sedation, PU/PD/PP, hepatic failure	Liver function monitoring is advisable
Potassium bromide	30–40 mg/kg q24h	PU/PD, vomiting, eosinophilic bronchopneumonia	Serum level monitoring
Clorazepate	3.75–7.5 mg/kg q6–12h	As diazepam	
Levetiracetam	10–20 mg/kg q8h	Inappetence, sedation, hypersalivation	
Gabapentin	5–20 mg/kg q6–12h	Sedation, ataxia	No clinical studies available
Zonisamide	5–10 mg/kg q12–24h	Sedation, inappetence, vomiting, diarrhea	
Pregabalin	1–2 mg/kg q12h	Sedation	No clinical studies available
Propentophyllin	5 mg/kg q12h		No clinical studies available
Taurine	100–400 mg/cat q24h		Inhibitory aminoacid
Topiramate	12.5–25 mg q8–12h	Sedation, inappetence	No clinical studies available

PU, polyuria; PD, polydipsia; PP, polyphagia.

Figure 3.6 Table of a review paper on feline epilepsy showing the references used for proving the validity of specific statements, in this case possible adverse effects of oral antiepileptic treatments for cats (Pakozdy, A., Halasz, P., & Klang, A. (2014). Epilepsy in cats: theory and practice. *Journal of Veterinary Internal Medicine*, **28**(2):255–263. © Wiley).

The peer-review process is usually performed by two or three professionals with experience in the area covered in the article. Yet, nobody is infallible, and even during the review process things can go past the reviewers and the article gets published in spite of some errors in analysis or interpretation. This unfortunately translates in the fact that, just because something is published, it does not mean that is good work, accurate, or true.

> Not everything that is published is scientific evidence.

So, if everything published cannot be considered scientific evidence, how do you decide what to use and what not? Review articles are a good place to start when you do not know much about a disease or condition. However, it is evident that the original studies (commonly known as research papers) are those used as references for all other types of articles and the ones that provide the scientific evidence for the practitioner. Remember, though, that just because some research was published, it does not mean that the research was correctly performed, reported, or interpreted. This is something the reader needs to evaluate.

References are used to show that a statement can be presented as a fact because someone proved it. Therefore, any statement that is presented as a fact should have be referenced. Most research papers will provide only one or two statements that can be referenced. The reason for this is that they study a specific question, such as "does treatment with a cream containing 1% hydrogen peroxide improve wound healing compared to using petrolatum?" (Toth *et al.* 2011), where the answer is either yes or no. For some studies, the answer may have some qualifiers. For example, in a study on the effect of gold bead implants on pain in dogs with osteoarthritis (Jaeger *et al.* 2005), the question was "does gold bead implantation reduce pain signs in dogs with osteoarthritis as assessed by their owners?" and the answer was "yes, in general, but more so in dogs up to 4 years old, than in older dogs." However, a broader question such as "is early neuter/spay in dogs associated with increased disease risk?" (Spain *et al.* 2004) will provide several answers, one for each specific disease that was studied, and therefore several referenced statements.

To reference a prevalence or an incidence, it is acceptable to quote recent papers (within 0–5 years). However, when an original idea or a statement is being quoted in an article, the first paper that presented that idea should be referenced; the original authors should be given appropriate credit for their discovery or idea.

> Any statement that is presented as a fact should be referenced.

Evaluation of a research paper

The general outline of a research paper includes, in this order, the following:
- Title
- Author names and affiliations
- Abstract or summary
- Introduction
- Materials and methods
- Results

- Discussion
- Conclusions
- References
- Acknowledgments

Abstract

Background: The risk of injuries is of major concern when keeping horses in groups and there is a need for a system to record external injuries in a standardised and simple way. The objective of this study, therefore, was to develop and validate a system for injury recording in horses and to test its reliability and feasibility under field conditions.

Methods: Injuries were classified into five categories according to severity. The scoring system was tested for intra- and inter-observer agreement as well as agreement with a "golden standard" (diagnosis established by a veterinarian). The scoring was done by 43 agricultural students who classified 40 photographs presented to them twice in a random order, 10 days apart. Attribute agreement analysis was performed using Kendall's coefficient of concordance (Kendall's W), Kendall's correlation coefficient (Kendall's τ) and Fleiss' kappa. The system was also tested on a sample of 100 horses kept in groups where injury location was recorded as well.

Results: Intra-observer agreement showed Kendall's W ranging from 0.94 to 0.99 and 86% of observers had kappa values above 0.66 (substantial agreement). Inter-observer agreement had an overall Kendall's W of 0.91 and the mean kappa value was 0.59 (moderate). Agreement for all observers versus the "golden standard" had Kendall's τ of 0.88 and the mean kappa value was 0.66 (substantial). The system was easy to use for trained persons under field conditions. Injuries of the more serious categories were not found in the field trial.

Conclusion: The proposed injury scoring system is easy to learn and use also for people without a veterinary education, it shows high reliability, and it is clinically useful. The injury scoring system could be a valuable tool in future clinical and epidemiological studies.

Figure 3.7 Summary of an original study (structured abstract) (Mejdell, C.M., Jorgensen, G.H., Rehn, T., Fremstad, K., Keeling, L., & Boe, K.E. (2010). Reliability of an injury scoring system for horses. *Acta Veterinaria Scandinavica*, **52**:68).

Titles are usually defined by the publishing journal to be of a certain length, and therefore some may indicate better than others what the article is about. *Author names and affiliations* are useful to track research interests, as well as to determine if the study in question was performed by a neutral third party or someone with vested interests in a study product.

The *abstract or summary*, which is what most people read (exclusively), should concisely and accurately summarize all other parts of the article (usually within a limit of 250 words). Nothing new should be presented in the abstract that is not mentioned within the article. However, it is impossible to summarize all findings in the constraint of the 250 words and, therefore, abstracts present filtered information, commonly sensationalized to attract the reader. People who only read the abstract walk away with a distorted understanding of the article as they do not evaluate the entire article to determine if the conclusions summarized in the abstract are warranted and legitimate. Sometimes, the abstract is formatted with section titles (structured abstract, Figure 3.7) and sometimes it is presented as a continuous paragraph (nonstructured abstract, Figure 3.8).

Abstracts present filtered information, commonly sensationalized to attract the reader.

Summary:

Sixteen toy breed dogs completed a parallel, 70-day two-period, cross-over design clinical study to determine the effect of a vegetable dental chew on gingivitis, halitosis, plaque, and calculus accumulations. The dogs were randomly assigned into two groups. During one study period the dogs were fed a non-dental dry diet only and during the second study period were fed the same dry diet supplemented by the daily addition of a vegetable dental chew. Daily administration of the dental chew was shown to reduce halitosis, as well as, significantly reduce gingivitis, plaque and calculus accumulation and therefore may play a significant role in the improvement of canine oral health over the long-term. **J Vet Dent 28 (4); 230–235, 2011**

Figure 3.8 Summary of an original study (nonstructured abstract) (Clarke, D.E., Kelman, M., & Perkins, N. (2011). Effectiveness of a vegetable dental chew on periodontal disease parameters in toy breed dogs. *Journal of Veterinary Dentistry*, **28**(4):230–235).

Example

An article that was looking into a possible relationship between antimicrobial use in food animals and antimicrobial resistance in bacteria isolated from humans (Spika *et al.* 1987) finishes its abstract with the sentence "We conclude that food animals are a major source of antimicrobial-resistant salmonella infections in humans and that these infections are associated with antimicrobial use on farms." However, this conclusion was never mentioned in the text. To warrant this conclusion, the authors should have measured antimicrobial use (which they did not), resistance to multiple antimicrobials (which they did not, they only evaluated chloramphenicol), in multiple food animals species (which they did not, they only studied cattle), and appropriately compare it with other "sources" of *Salmonella* infection (which they did not). Additionally, the data presented in the results show that the major factor that was significantly associated with chloramphenicol-resistant *Salmonella* infections in humans was the use of tetracycline or penicillin in those humans in the previous 30 days of the study. Yet this study continues to be the one cited as proof of a link between food animals and resistance in bacteria isolated from humans (Table 3.1).

Table 3.1 Reported association strength of chloramphenicol-resistant *Salmonella* infections in humans with different studied risk factors.

	Patients		Controls		OR	P-value
	%	N	%	N		
Antibiotic use <30 days (tetracyclines, penicillins)	24	45	2	88	19.6	<0.001
Ground beef <1 week	98	43	85	85	7.9	0.052
"Nibbled" on raw meat	15	41	3	70	4.7	<0.02
Hamburger from producer A	20	N/A	3	N/A	12.7	<0.008

Data compiled from text in Spika, J.S., Waterman, S.H., Hoo, G.W., St Louis, M.E., Pacer, R.E., James, S.M., Bissett, M.L., Mayer, L.W., Chiu, J.Y., & Hall, B. (1987). Chloramphenicol-resistant *Salmonella* Newport traced through hamburger to dairy farms. A major persisting source of human salmonellosis in California. *The New England Journal of Medicine*, **316**:565–570.
N/A, not applicable.

The *introduction* should include information about what is known about the disease or condition at the time of redaction of the article. It should include a thorough literature review that is summarized to give a good but concise overview. The objectives of the study are always presented in the last paragraph of the introduction. Objectives should be concise and measurable so that the outcomes can be analyzed.

The *materials and methods* section should detail the study in enough detail to allow anyone who reads the article to be able to duplicate the study exactly as it was originally done and, therefore, to obtain similar results. Most important in this section are the inclusion and exclusion criteria (case definition) to determine eligible and noneligible animals, as well as the definition of the control group for comparison.

The *results* section includes text, tables, and graphs that summarize only objective findings of the study. This means that no interpretations of the results should be included here. Initially, the overall descriptive statistics of the study groups should be presented, which is later scrutinized in specific layers (strata) such as animal age, breed, and gender. This is usually presented as the first table of a research paper. Also, animals leaving the study need to be mentioned, and according to the circumstances of the study described, so that the reader can evaluate the impact of losing those animals on the overall study. After that, the content of the different tables and graphs will vary from article to article to portray the most important results. Secondary results are usually presented in the text only. **Statistical significance** is information (*P* value) that is provided to allow the reader to evaluate the validity of the results.

The discussion and conclusion sections are often presented together, but they are different things. In the *discussion*, the authors will explain what they think the results mean, and show if their results agree with similar studies previously published, and if not, they will argue the reasons why they think they do not agree. In the *conclusion*, the authors will decide what the results mean (**biological significance**) to them based on their previous experience and their circumstances and if they could answer the research question. This is called the internal validity of a study, the ability to produce a conclusion based on the results. Additionally, the authors will make potential conclusions (inferences) that may be applicable to other populations. These inferences need to take into account the type of population and circumstances surrounding the study, so they can truly be applicable to other populations. This is called the external validity of a study.

Example

Results from a study performed on lions in the Serengeti in Tanzania (Africa) will likely not be applicable to indoor cats living in Hong Kong or lynx living in Alaska due to differences in ecosystems, pollution, and climate.

Authors should detail in the discussion if there were any pitfalls and what can be done in the future to prevent those pitfalls or to improve the reliability of the study. It is important to note that the conclusions drawn by the authors may not coincide with those reached by all readers, as they may have different experience, background, or interests. Examples of this are commonly found in studies of new treatment options that only provide marginal improvement over previous options.

Example

A study on the effect of chemotherapy of advanced hemangiosarcoma in dogs (Dervisis *et al.* 2011) concluded in the abstract that "the DAV (doxorubicin, dacarbacin and vincristine) combination appears to offer clinical responses and may prolong survival in dogs with advanced-stage HAS," while in the text the conclusion is more moderate: "the DAV protocol appears to be active against advanced-stage, non-cutaneous hemangiosarcoma in the dog." The results of the study showed that with a treatment cycle duration of 21 days, median time to death of dogs was 125 days. This in itself may seem OK. But when we take into account that dogs had to visit the hospital three times in each treatment cycle (21-day period) to undergo treatment that required some drug administrations over 8 h with IV catheters, sedation and preparation for drug administration, and that several of these drugs had toxic side effects severe enough to require dose restriction, to allow 50% of them to live no more than 4 months, many practitioners would conclude that this is not an effective treatment. It is important to note, however, that this study may give some ideas of new directions of study in the treatment of cancer that was not possible until now. Therefore, the conclusions can vary depending on the specific interest of the person interpreting the results.

Data presentation in the results

The way the data are presented can make a huge difference in the perception of the results by most readers, especially when using graphs. Most people are driven by visual cues and, therefore, certain visual representations of the data can induce erroneous perceptions of the results. A typical misleading graph uses a truncated axis to show a visually large difference between two or more groups that are being compared. This issue is more common and intentional in the lay literature (e.g., product advertisements) than in the peer-reviewed literature. However, being aware of it will make spotting these issues easier and result in more accurate interpretation.

Example

Consider the two graphs in Figures 3.9 and 3.10, which visually depict the number of donkeys that recovered or died in a study about the effects of impaction colic in donkeys (Cox *et al.* 2007). They both represent exactly the same data. The only difference between them is the range of the *Y*-axis; on the left we have a range of 48–52%, while on the right we have 0–100%. Even using the same colors in the graphs, the information drawn visually is completely different. Using the left graph as reference, it appears that many more donkeys with impaction colic died than with other types of colic, when in reality there was no difference between the groups.

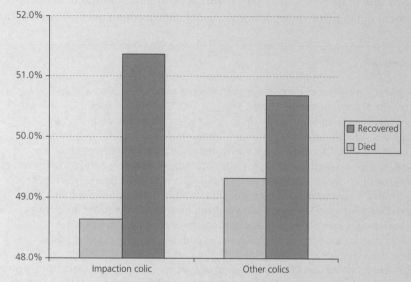

Figure 3.9 Misrepresented data (Cox, R., Proudman, C.J., Trawford, A.F., Burden, F., & Pinchbeck, G.L. (2007). Epidemiology of impaction colic in donkeys in the UK. *BMC Veterinary Research*, **3**:1–11).

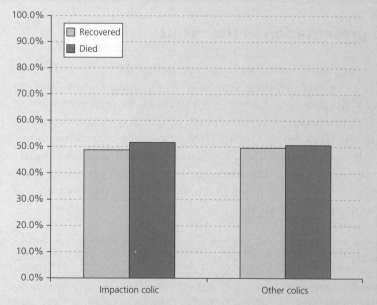

Figure 3.10 Appropriate data presentation (Cox, R., Proudman, C.J., Trawford, A.F., Burden, F., & Pinchbeck, G.L. (2007). Epidemiology of impaction colic in donkeys in the UK. *BMC Veterinary Research*, **3**:1–11).

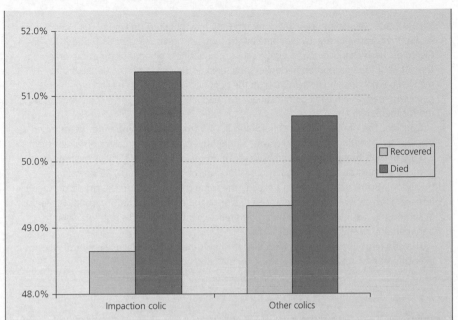

Figure 3.11 Effect of color on data presentation leading to possible misinterpretation (Cox, R., Proudman, C.J., Trawford, A.F., Burden, F., & Pinchbeck, G.L. (2007). Epidemiology of impaction colic in donkeys in the UK. *BMC Veterinary Research*, **3**:1–11).

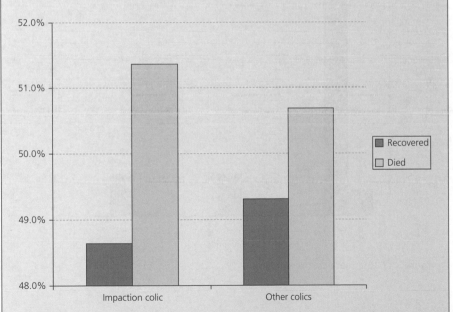

Figure 3.12 Effect of color on data presentation helping toward correct interpretation (Cox, R., Proudman, C.J., Trawford, A.F., Burden, F., & Pinchbeck, G.L. (2007). Epidemiology of impaction colic in donkeys in the UK. *BMC Veterinary Research*, **3**:1–11).

Now consider the difference in interpretation you may obtain from Figures 3.11 and 3.12. Again, they represent exactly the same information as shown in Figures 3.9 and 3.10, but the colors have changed. Do you get a sense of uneasiness when looking at the graph on the left about the proportion of donkeys that died or the proportion of donkeys that recovered when looking at the graph on the right? It is likely due to having grown up perceiving dark as a meaning of "caution" or "danger." Now imagine a color chart using red for these data.

Consider the graphs in Figures 3.13 and 3.14 from a study comparing the number of calvings, resulting in stillborn calves, singleton calves, or twin calves obtained from a dairy herd in three groups of cows (*X*-axis): normal calving (<285 days gestation), induced parturition (at 285 days of gestation), or long gestation (>285 days of gestation). Both graphs represent exactly the same data; however, the graph on the left seems to show a huge difference in favor of the normal gestation group, while the graph on the right seems to show no difference in stillbirths and singleton calvings between any of the three groups.

The difference is that the graph on the left shows the raw data (actual count of calvings in each group of cows), while the graph on the right shows the percentage.

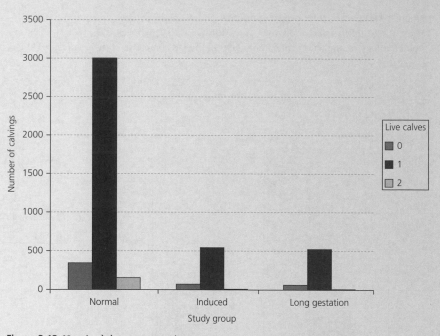

Figure 3.13 Nominal data presentation.

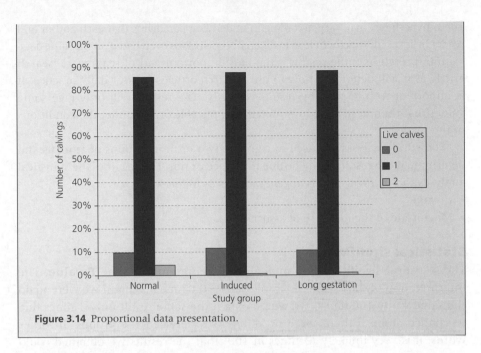

Figure 3.14 Proportional data presentation.

In summary, to avoid misinterpretation of graphical data, it is imperative to define each axis appropriately and in detail. The X-axis tells us *what* is being presented and the Y-axis gives us the clue as to *how* things are being presented.

Interpretation of results

By far, the most important part of any study is the interpretation of the results. Conclusions drawn from a study should be warranted by the results. If a pattern is detected, there may be one or more hypotheses to explain why the pattern exists.

Example

Provided is an excerpt of a quote by Sir Arthur Eddington (1958) in his *Philosophy of Physical Science* that vividly represents the conundrums of research:

> *Let us suppose that an ichthyologist is exploring the life of the ocean. He casts a net into the water and brings up a fishy assortment. Surveying his catch, he proceeds in the usual manner of a scientist to systematise what it reveals. He arrives at two generalisations: (1) no sea-creature is less than two inches long and (2) all sea-creatures have gills.*

The conclusions of the ichthyologist are warranted by his observations, but we know that both of his conclusions are not true. Had he used a fishing net with smaller holes, he would probably change both of his conclusions. We know that his conclusions are not true because other scientists who have studied life in the ocean with methods other than a fishing net have found sea creatures that are smaller than two inches and sea creatures that do not have gills.

These hypotheses may vary according to underlying paradigms that each author and reader believes in, which can lead to different conclusions even based on the same data.

Interpretation of the results is the most important part of reading a research article as it will determine how to use research articles in your daily practice. It is important to interpret the results correctly. The results will only give some values that then need to be interpreted as applicable or not under the conditions of the reader.

Statistical analyses are used to compare two or more groups of animals and determine if the results could be due to chance or not. The result of the statistical analyses can be divided in two general parts as follows:

- *P*-value
- Magnitude of the measure of association

Statistical significance

The statistical significance of an analysis is represented by the **P-value**. The interpretation of the P-value is as follows: $P = 0.03$ means that if we were to do the same study 100 times, we would obtain the same result only 3 times due to chance alone if there were no differences between the groups. In other words, it is very unlikely (3 times in 100) that the results we obtained could happen by chance and not due to a true association of the study variable and the outcome.

Notice that we do not refer to "random events" as the word random implies something very specific to epidemiologists (see Chapter 4).

Most researchers use a level of significance of 5% to determine if their results are statistically significant or not. However, this value is not written in stone anywhere and for some studies with limited availability of study subjects, it is perfectly acceptable to use a level of significance of 10%. Whatever the level of significance, the P-value has the same interpretation, depending on whether it is above or below the level of significance established in the materials and methods (before the study is started). Using a level of significance of 5%, the interpretation is as follows:

- P-value ≤5% means that there is equal or less than 5% probability that the results obtained in the study were due to chance alone. Because of this small probability of the results being due to chance alone, it is concluded that the difference measured between the studied groups has to be real, and therefore the studied variable is considered to be associated with the outcome.
- P-value >5% (even if it is 5.1%) is interpreted as though the difference between the groups is likely due to chance, probably meaning that there is another risk factor that has not been identified yet and needs to be studied further (see Chapter 2).

In graphs, statistical significance is commonly shown with the help of error bars to represent the standard error of the mean of the represented data. If the error bars overlap, the difference between two groups is not statistically significant (Figure 3.15), while if the error bars do not overlap, the difference is statistically significant.

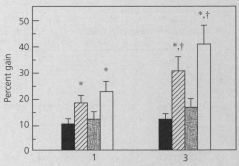

Mean (SEM) percentage weight gain in four groups of cats one
and three months after they were neutered or left intact (■ = sexually intact
male, ◩ = neutered male, ▦ = sexually intact female, ☐ = spayed female).
* Significantly different from sexually intact groups of same gender ($P < 0.05$),
† Significantly different from one month after neutering ($P < 0.05$)

Figure 3.15 Use of error bars for the representation of the standard error of the mean
(Fettman, M.J., Stanton, C.A., Banks, L.L., Hamar, D.W., Johnson, D.E., Hegstad, R.L., &
Johnston, S. (1997). Effects of neutering on bodyweight, metabolic rate and glucose
tolerance of domestic cats. *Research in Veterinary Science*, **62**:131–136. © Elsevier).

Example

Consider the graph (Figure 3.15) presented from a study on the effect of neutering (risk
factor) on weight gain in cats (Fettman *et al.* 1997). Error bars are used to represent the
standard error of the mean, and it is easy therefore to see which groups are statistically
different and which ones are not. This interpretation is also facilitated by the use of the
marks atop the groups that are different.

Statistical significance depends largely on sample size for each group: the larger
the sample size, the smaller the *P*-value that can be achieved. Therefore, studies
with large sample sizes tend to achieve good *P*-values and tend to be more credible
than studies with small sample sizes, where chance may have more possibility
to intervene. However, it has little to do with the difference obtained in the
outcome when the study variable is applied to a population.

Example

Consider the table presented from a study on early spay/neuter (risk factor) by Spain *et al.*
2004 (Figure 3.16). According to this table, most of the studied outcome variables were
significantly associated with early spay/neuter as indicated by the small *P*-values (<5%
or 0.05). However, the biological significance of many of these outcomes is minor. For
example, is it worthy to perform early spay/neuter when the desired outcome is to avoid
barking that annoys household members? The *P*-value indicates that the result is highly
significant (statistically), meaning that the difference is not due to chance alone and we
can rely on it. However, the parameter (OR = 1.08) indicates that the difference is only 8%
between early and late spay/neuter. So, is it worth it for that purpose?

Behavior	Age at gonadectomy (mo)	Dogs with behavior (%)	Odds ratio	95% CI	Overall P value
Aggression towards household members[a]	<5.5 ≥5.5	29.0 21.5	1.32 1.0	1.05, 2.10 NA	0.02
Barking that bothered household members[a,b]	Continuous	34.2	1.08[c]	1.02, 1.12	<0.01
Barking or growling at visitors[a,b]	Continuous	65.4	1.08[c]	1.02, 1.13	<0.01
Escaping from home (serious problem)	Continuous	9.6	0.93[c]	0.87, 0.98	<0.01
Noise phobia[b]	Continuous	52.6	1.04[c]	1.01, 1.08	<0.01
Separation anxiety	<5.5 ≥5.5	14.2 18.7	0.72 1.0	0.55, 0.94 NA	0.02
Sexual behaviors[b]	Continuous	27.3	1.05[c]	1.01, 1.09	<0.01
Urination when frightened[c]	<5.5 ≥5.5	9.4 12.3	0.74 1.0	0.54, 1.01 NA	0.06

[a]Male dogs only. [b]Not significant ($P > 0.05$) when considered a serious problem. [c]Odds ratio/1-month decrease in age at gonadectomy.

Figure 3.16 Behavioral conditions associated with early gonadectomy in 1659 dogs (Spain, C.V., Scarlett, J.M., & Houpt, K.A. (2004). Long-term risks and benefits of early-age gonadectomy in dogs. *Journal of the American Veterinary Medical Association*, **224**(3): 380–387. © AVMA).

Biological significance

Biological significance is represented by the magnitude of the measure of association in the statistical analyses. Each clinician or researcher will decide if the magnitude is biologically significant to them or not. No level of statistical significance is more important than biological significance.

Example

Assume a difference in resting heart rate (outcome variable) of 10% between horses that are exercised for 3 h/day versus horses that are not regularly exercised (risk factor). This translates into a difference of approximately 4–5 beats per minute. Is this biologically significant to you? In other words, is it worth to exercise the horses 3 h/day to lower the heart rate by 4–5 beats per minute? You have to decide that.

Now consider, for example (completely fictitious), a difference of 10% in the incidence of osteosarcoma (outcome variable) in Chihuahuas that are carried in purses if the cell phone is also carried in the purse versus no cell phone in the purse (risk factor). Is this biologically significant? Is it worth to the owners not carrying the cell phone in the same purse as the Chihuahua to reduce osteosarcoma incidence by 10%? You and the owners decide.

Interesting to note here is that each owner you interact with on a daily basis is evaluating the biological significance of everything you present to him/her. In other words, they will question every single recommendation you make in light of its worthiness in terms of cost, return on investment, effort, animal well-being, etc. Animal owners understand biological significance.

Biological significance answers the question of "whether it is worth to do X to obtain Y."

My hope is that after applying the knowledge in this chapter, you will realize that you can determine if a study warrants the conclusions that are published or not and whether you can use that information to help your patients.

4 Study designs

The methodology behind a study is very important to determine whether the results could be biased and whether the results can be extrapolated to other groups of animals.

Example

Assume a researcher conducts a study of the effect of weight and body condition score (BCS) on skeletal integrity and arthritis using neutered Beagles (a typical research breed) in the range of 2–5 years of age. A clinician reads the study and tries to apply the results to a pregnant 7-year-old St. Bernard bitch. Is this reasonable given the differences in bone physiology (i.e., calcium and phosphorus) of a neutered dog and a pregnant bitch? Could the results of a study performed only on Beagles be applicable to other dog breeds?

Study designs can be classified according to several characteristics. A basic classification separates the studies that observe without imposing any intervention on the animals called **observational studies** and the ones that impose some type of intervention on the animals or **clinical trials**. By definition, clinical trials are **prospective studies**, where the timeline of the study begins with animals that are not exposed to the risk factors under investigation and before the outcome can be observed or measured. The opposite are **retrospective studies**, where the timeline of the study begins after the exposure factors have had their effect and the outcome is already observed or measured. In other words, they go backward. Additionally, study designs may require statistical analysis to compare risk factors and their effect on an outcome, in which case they are termed **analytical studies**, or they can merely describe findings in a population, in which

---

Practical Clinical Epidemiology for the Veterinarian, First Edition. Aurora Villarroel.
© 2015 John Wiley & Sons, Inc. Published 2015 by John Wiley & Sons, Inc.
Companion website: www.wiley.com/go/villarroel/epidemiology

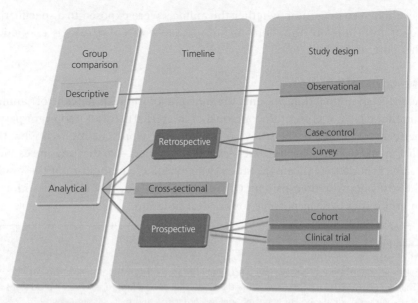

Figure 4.1 Types of study designs according to different characteristics.

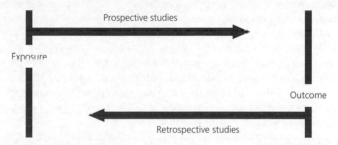

Figure 4.2 Comparison of flow of information in prospective and retrospective studies.

case they are termed **descriptive studies**. An overall view of the different study designs and how they relate to each other is presented (Figure 4.1), and the flows of information direction are presented in graphical form in Figure 4.2.

> A good study design will allow better statistical analyses.

Retrospective studies

The most important characteristic of retrospective studies is that all animals start with a known status of disease and are separated into the control or study group based on disease status: disease-free or affected. The cornerstone of retrospective studies is the existence of records about whether there has been exposure to potential risk factors and the timing of both the exposure and the outcome. Records are evaluated back to a specific time or amount of time and are evaluated to determine whether the animals were exposed to a specific risk factor or not. Therefore, the main outcome of **case–control studies** is association with a potential risk factor.

Case–control studies

A "case" is an animal that presents the outcome of interest. A "control" animal is one that does not present the outcome of interest. The most important part is to perfectly discriminate the study groups; in other words, define well what the inclusion and exclusion criteria are—even if not perfect—so that anyone can use the same criteria to replicate the study or to evaluate whether or not the results of the study apply to their patient. Obviously, it would be best if the definition of each group is as close as possible to the ideal situation.

Example

For example, in a study that evaluated possible risk factors for diabetes mellitus in cats (Sallander *et al.* 2012), a case was defined as a cat that had at least one of ten typical signs of diabetes (polydipsia, polyuria, polyphagia, weight loss, abnormal gait, lethargy, vomiting, weakness, anorexia, or coma) as well as fasting hyperglycemia (>10 mmol/l) and high fructosamine levels (>400 μmol/l). A control was defined as a cat that was in the same database but had been seen in the hospital for a regular health visit or prophylaxis. Control cats were matched by age.

It is apparent that the definition of the groups is not necessarily ideal, but it is clear and it can be replicated. A more detailed definition for a case in this study would have required at least 5 of the 10 typical signs of diabetes, while the control group could have been more tightly matched as cats that had those same characteristics at the same time as the case cat, and possibly eating the same type of food (Figure 4.3), to eliminate some additional risk factors that could affect the interpretation of results.

Food item	Cases (n=20)			Controls (n=20)		
	Proportion yes (%)[a]	Proportion (% of total intake, DM/d)[a, b]		Proportion yes (%)[a]	Proportion (% of total intake, DM/d)[a, b]	
		Median	Min-max		Median	Min-max
Dry foods	85	44	0–100	85	79*	0–100
Canned foods	70	48	0–100	75	20	0–100
Table foods	65	10	5–30	80	6	1–20
Vitamins/minerals	40	—		25	—	
Treats	10	—		20	—	

[a]Fishers exact test significant at *P≤0.05.
[b]To calculated the proportion of food given (g dry matter/d), the dry matter has been estimated to 90 and 20% in dry and canned/table foods, respectively.

Figure 4.3 Comparison of diets in cats with diabetes mellitus and age-matched controls (Sallander, M., Eliasson, J., & Hedhammar, A. (2012). Prevalence and risk factors for the development of diabetes mellitus in Swedish cats. *Acta Veterinaria Scandinavica*, **54**:61).

It may be confusing for some the fact that "control" can be used to describe an animal from the point of view of the outcome (i.e., does not present the outcome of interest) or from the point of view of the risk factor (i.e., is not exposed to the risk factor). In both cases however, notice that it refers to the animals that are not exposed or do not present the outcome, so they represent the group to be used as baseline comparison for the treatment or case group. Also notice that the definition of a "case" here is in balance with the definition presented in Chapter 2.

Limitations of case–control studies

Because they begin after the outcome has been detected, it is impossible to determine if the risk factors found to be associated with the outcome are in fact a cause or simply associated (see Chapter 5). Another major limitation is the need for very detailed records or running the risk of having recall bias when these records are not in place and exposure is "remembered."

Advantages of case–control studies

Because we know the outcome when we start the study, it is easier to ensure adequate sample size in both groups, and fewer animals need to be enrolled in the study because it is not necessary to wait until a case occurs, especially when working with diseases that have low incidence. This makes case–control studies less expensive compared with prospective studies.

Example

A study about a disease that has an incidence of 1 in 1000 animal-days would require evaluating at least 1000 animal-days to observe one case if it were a prospective study. This could be mathematically accomplished in scenarios anywhere in between the following two extremes:
- Enrolling one animal in the study and observing it over 1000 days
- Enrolling 1000 animals and observing them for 1 day
  This would be required to obtain a single case. However, a retrospective study can look for cases that have already happened, and select several and study them backward in time compared with control animals to determine possible risk factors by identifying exposures that were more common in the case group than in the control group.

Surveys

Surveys are a powerful method to collect a lot of information from one source and are commonly used for retrospective studies. However, using the right questions, surveys can be used for other types of studies. Because of this, the surveys have been abused and have become a nuisance in some instances, leading to incomplete or useless information in that it cannot be analyzed properly. Simply think back of the latest survey you have answered as we cover some of the main characteristics.

There are entire books written about how to conduct surveys appropriately, so we will not cover this in depth. However, it is worth listing some key recommendations to take into account when conducting and evaluating a survey and are as follows:
- Questions should have objective and very concrete answers that cover all possible answers and do not overlap between answers.

Example

Imagine the question is "where do you keep your horse?," and the answers provided to check in the survey are "on pasture," "in a barn," "in a horse stable," and "others." Some respondents may feel torn between choosing a barn and a stable if there are only a few horses in the facility or no strict definitions of each type of facility. Additionally, horses allowed on pasture part-time would not fit into any of the categories provided and their owners may decide to select the "others" answer, which may bias the results when, for example, looking at parasite exposure through dew on grass. A better question with this intention in mind would be "do you allow your horse out on pasture in the early morning or late evening when there is dew on the grass?" with the most simple answers "yes" and "no," or more complicated answers that can attempt to semi-quantify risk using "never," "once a week or less," "2–4 days per week," and "more than 4 days per week."

- Open-ended questions should be avoided; a choice of answers allows better analysis because it provides the same answer for each participant as opposed to "similar answers."

Example

The answer to the question "is the dog white?" is either yes or no. However, if to get the same information we ask "what color is the dog?" along with all other possible colors that are not even close to white, we may get some people answering "off-white," "cream," and others. It is truly amazing to read some of the answers you get to open-ended questions!

Questions that only have the option of being answered as yes/no are the best types of questions. If at any point, there is the potential of answering "maybe" or "it depends," then the question should be reformulated to allow a simple yes/no answer.

- Questions that ask more than one idea or could have compounded answers should be avoided.
- Terms that may be open to interpretation such as "maybe," "often," "sometimes," "regularly," and "appropriately" should avoided both in the question and the answers.

Example

In the question "are horse stalls cleaned regularly and appropriately?," what exactly is the meaning of "regularly" and "appropriately"? A barn that is cleaned once a year is cleaned on a regular interval, and yet it would likely not be considered appropriate. And should the answer to this question be "yes" or "no" if we think it is appropriate but it is not regular?

- Answers that chunk information in categories a priori should be avoided, asking instead for numbers and making the appropriate categories during the analysis. Numerical data cannot be restored if only categorical data are recorded.
- The number of questions should be kept to the absolute minimum necessary, preventing fatigue and loss of interest by the respondents, which will likely translate into nonreliable information.
- A logical flow of questions avoids confusion in the respondents.

Example

A study on dystocia in Boxers (Linde Forsberg and Persson 2007) used a survey to gather their information (Figure 4.4). Questions 1 and 2 of the survey seem to cover all possible options. However, in Question 3, the authors combined X-ray and ultrasound examination together, making the answer of "dead fetus/fetuses" nonapplicable to X-ray examination, while other answers were vague (i.e., how many were a few pups). The survey was only one page long, which made it easy to fill and likely improved the response rate (it was not reported in the study).

Whelping survey
Breeder:
Litter:
Date of birth:

1. **Was veterinary help needed during the whelping**   □ yes   □ no   if no, continue to question 7.

2. **If veterinary help was needed, was the reason**
   □ Straining never started
   □ Straining was weak
   □ Straining ceased after one/a few of the pups were born. No. of pups delivered ....
   □ Strong strainings but no pup was born
   □ Other reason ....

3. **If x-ray/ultrasound examination was done, was the following found**
   □ Malposition of fetus
   □ Only 1 or few pups
   □ Dead fetus/fetuses
   □ Many pups/large litter
   □ Other findings ....

Figure 4.4 Extract of a survey on dystocia in Boxers (Linde Forsberg, F.C., & Persson, G. (2007). A survey of dystocia in the boxer breed. *Acta Veterinaria Scandinavica*, **49**:8).

Limitations of surveys

Like other retrospective studies, surveys that look at historical information have the potential of recall bias; respondents may filter the answers intentionally or unintentionally (they simply forgot). Another major limitation is the likely inaccuracy of some answers due to simple misinterpretation of the question or because none of the categorical answers really fits well, so the respondent chooses the closest match.

Example

In a study we performed using a survey on the reasons why veterinarians decided to enter rural practice (Villarroel *et al.* 2010), there were disparate interpretations of what constituted rural practice. Most respondents (93.4%) defined rural practice to be associated with agricultural communities, but not all. This means that 16.6% of our respondents were defining the outcome in a different way and, therefore, results of this group may not be directly comparable with the others. We could have established a detailed definition of what rural practice meant to us, but we were indeed interested in what the respondents' interpretation was. For analysis purposes, to ensure direct comparability, one option is to analyze results only in the group that interpreted rural practice the same way.

  In that same study, we asked when veterinarians had developed their interest in rural practice, and the answers were categorized according to the different levels of education throughout the years: before eighth grade, in high school, during undergraduate school, during vet school, or in graduate school. We included an "other" category for flexibility, which 2.2% of the respondents marked. Our intention was to establish at what age their interest had developed, but the categories we established did not fit someone who developed their interest for rural practice during the 1–2 years they worked at a farm after undergraduate school before deciding they would even become a veterinarian.

Advantages of surveys

They allow collection of vast amount of information and exploration of multiple risk factors at once. Because they do not require the use of measurements on any animals, surveys tend to not be as expensive as other studies.

Cross-sectional studies

These studies are very common in the veterinary literature. **Cross-sectional studies** measure the risk factors and the outcome in any given animal at the same time. The study itself may expand multiple days, weeks, months, or even years to collect enough data, but the key feature is that an individual animal is sampled only once and both the risk factors and the outcomes are measured at the same time. Because of this, it is not possible to draw conclusions about causal relationship (see Chapter 5), but these types of studies are well suited to determine prevalence of a condition and to identify possible risk factors that are highly associated with the outcome and should be looked into with more detail in prospective studies to establish if they are, in fact, causal or not.

Example

In a study of gastric ulcers in race horses (Vatistas *et al.* 1999), the authors studied the relationship between the presence of gastric ulcers and several possible risk factors. In the experimental protocol (Figure 4.5), they report that they obtained a blood sample at the same time that they performed the endoscopy. Therefore, the outcome (gastric ulceration score) was measured at the same time as all the possible risk factor variables studied (hematologic values), and thus it is impossible to tell whether the ulcers appeared before or after any possible changes in hematologic values.

Experimental protocol

Two hundred and two Thoroughbred horses in active race training were selected from trainers willing to participate in the study by their attending veterinarians. Horses had to have been in active race training at the race track for at least 2 months prior to endoscopic examination. Horses that were not in active race training due to lameness and/or illness were excluded.

Prior to endoscopic examination, the trainer, in conjunction with the attending veterinarian, was requested to complete a questionnaire covering the previous one month, which included: body condition; appetite; disposition; presence of lameness and training expectations (Table 1).

Other more objective criteria included: class in which the horse raced (although the duration between the last race and the endoscopic examination was not recorded); administration of nonsteroidal anti-inflammatory agents (NSAIDs); administration of frusemide; and occurrence of one or more episodes of colic or diarrhoea over the previous one month (Table 2).

Venous blood samples were obtained at the time of endoscopy for haematological and biochemical examination; and values used as another determinant of the health of the horse.

Figure 4.5 Experimental protocol for a study of gastric ulcers in race horses (Vatistas, N.J., Snyder, J.R., Carlson, G., Johnson, B., Arthur, R.M., Thurmond, M., Zhou, H., & Lloyd, K.L. (1999). Cross-sectional study of gastric ulcers of the squamous mucosa in thoroughbred racehorses. *Equine Veterinary Journal, Supplement,* **29**:34–39. © Wiley).

Limitations of cross-sectional studies

When population dynamics are ignored, discriminated, not well known, or not understood, the group of animals selected for sampling may not be representative of the entire population. It is not possible to establish if there is a causal relationship between the potential risk factors and the outcome because it is not possible to establish which was present first (see temporal association in Chapter 5), unless it is a genetically determined characteristic such as gender or breed. Cross-sectional studies often use some type of survey, which has its own limitations, as previously described.

> **Example**
>
> A study that looked at potential stressors related to human interaction in spotted hyenas in Kenya (Van Meter *et al.* 2009) specifically excluded adult males that were born within the studied clans because they reportedly have different behavior and physiology than immigrant males. In this case, the exclusion of this group of animals may have biased the results, making them not representative of the entire population.

Advantages of cross-sectional studies

They allow exploration of multiple risk factors at once, especially those that are genetically fixed such as gender and breed. When not using surveys as part of their data collection process, they avoid the potential for recall bias; data are measured in real time.

Prospective studies

These studies are also known as **longitudinal studies** in contrast to the cross-sectional studies described earlier. The most important characteristic of these studies is that all animals start free of disease and are separated into the study or control group based on exposure to a specific risk factor. Animals are observed for a specific amount of time and are evaluated to determine whether the outcome occurs in them or not. Therefore, the main outcome of cohort studies is incidence of disease.

Prospective studies allow the control of certain factors that could be considered confounding variables. They also allow good discrimination between groups using mutually exclusive characteristics so that there is no possible overlapping or potential for misclassification. For this, it is absolutely critical to define specific inclusion and exclusion criteria to perfectly discriminate between study groups.

Cohort studies

A **cohort** is a group of animals that share the same timeline, commonly the start of the study period. In cohort studies, a group of animals is followed over time to calculate the incidence of disease and potential risk factors (Figure 4.6). More than one cohort can be observed to determine whether the outcome has a different incidence in either of the groups, which may provide inferences about seasonality of a disease. Cohort studies are the quintessential observational studies where there is no intervention and nature is allowed to run its course. However, they are not commonly reported in the veterinary literature anymore because they are expensive and unpredictable. With a similar budget, it is possible to control the exposure and run a clinical trial. Cohort studies remain one of the best options for wild populations where human intervention would not be feasible or warranted.

Breed	Observational periods					
	7 weeks to 3 months	3 to 4 months	4 to 6 months	6 to 12 months	12 to 18 months	18 to 25 months
LEO	19/209	17/194	19/181	12/153	6/131	4/110
	9.1%	**8.8%**	**10.5%**	**7.8%**	**4.6%**	**3.6%**
	(5.9–13.8)	(5.5–13.6)	(6.8–15.8)	(4.5–13.2)	(2.1–9.6)	(1.4–9.0)
NF	9/137	2/129	1/123	0/100	2/85	1/60
	6.6%	**1.6%**	**0.8%**	**0%**	**2.3%**	**1.7%**
	(3.5–12.0)	(0.4–5.5)	(0.1–4.5)	(0.0–3.6)	(0.6–8.2)	(0.3–8.9)
LR	11/148	13/144	10/140	7/122	5/87	7/90
	7.4%	**9.0%**	**7.1%**	**5.7%**	**5.7%**	**7.8%**
	(4.2–12.8)	(5.4–14.8)	(3.9–12.6)	(2.8–11.4)	(2.5–12.8)	(3.8–15.2)
IW	2/81	5/79	5/70	4/55	2/45	0/34
	2.5%	**6.3%**	**7.1%**	**7.3%**	**4.4%**	**0%**
	(0.7–8.6)	(2.7–14.0)	(3.1–15.7)	(2.9–17.3)	(1.2–14.8)	(0.0–10.3)
Total	41/575	37/546	35/514	23/430	15/348	12/294
	7.1%	**6.8%**	**6.8%**	**5.3%**	**4.3%**	**4.1%**
	(5.3–9.5)	(5.0–9.2)	(4.9–9.3)	(3.6–7.9)	(2.6–7.0)	(2.4–7.0)

The study period is divided into six different observational periods, according to the given observational ages. Incidence risks are reported as percentages with 95% confidence intervals in brackets, with the number of episodes of vomiting in the numerator and the total number of reports retrieved at the observational ages as denominator. Leonberger (LEO), Newfoundland (NF), Labrador retriever (LR), and Irish wolfhound (IW).

Figure 4.6 Incidence risk of vomiting in dogs in different observational periods in a cohort study (Saevik, B.K., Skancke, E.M., & Trangerud, C. (2012). A longitudinal study on diarrhoea and vomiting in young dogs of four large breeds. *Acta Veterinaria Scandinavica*, **54**:8).

Limitations of cohort studies

They can quickly become expensive studies as it is difficult to estimate how many animals will develop the outcome, or how long it will take to develop that outcome. Additionally, it is common to lose animals to follow-up because they move outside of the study area, they are sold to another owner that doesn't want to participate in the study or who doesn't follow guidelines appropriately, the animals may acquire a disease or condition that is incompatible with the study or they die for reasons unrelated to the condition under study.

Example

Assume a study looking at risk factors for cub survival among free-ranging African lions in the savanna. A **cohort study** design would imply identifying pregnant lions and determining exactly when they gave birth and how many cubs they had without intervening (as this may alter the results if the dam became aggressive toward the cubs or accidentally stepped on them due to stress). Then each cub would have to be followed for a predetermined amount of time to note whether it succumbed to the environment or survived. If during the study, while tracking some of the lions, the investigator were to run over one of the cubs with his Jeep and kill it, would this death be considered as a nonsurvival for the purposes of the study or would this cub be eliminated from the study after so much time and effort?

Advantages of cohort studies

They are the best option to study disease incidence, although they will become prohibitively expensive when working with disease with very low incidence (as many animals need to be enrolled in the study to observe one with the outcome).

Clinical trials

They are also called field trials and are prospective studies in which one group of animals is exposed in a controlled manner to a potential risk factor (study group), while another group is consciously kept away from that same exposure (control group). Clinical trials are experiments conducted to evaluate the effect of an intervention on the outcome and require the use of statistical analysis to compare effects between groups. They are by far the most common study design in the modern veterinary literature.

The main differences between clinical trials and cohort studies, the two types of prospective studies, are (i) that clinical trials apply the potential risk factors in a controlled manner to the study group while in cohort studies the risk factors happen naturally and are simply observed and (ii) that clinical trials can specify inclusion and exclusion criteria while cohort studies may be less clear-cut in their exposures.

It is important to detail the design of the field trial in a manner that would allow any reader to exactly duplicate the same experiment. This is easily accomplished by showing a diagram of the flow of actions such as selection process, treatment applications, samples taken, and measurements taken as shown in Figure 4.7. Diagrams are also very helpful to establish the timeline of a protocol, especially when there are multiple interventions (Figure 4.8).

Clinical trials are based on the definition of a research question called the research or study hypothesis. Commonly this question is phrased as "evaluating the difference in (insert whatever you want here) between the study group and the control group." So, the study hypothesis is phrased as the presence of a difference. The statistical analyses, however, are commonly based on disproving the **null hypothesis** that there is no difference between the groups. Therefore, when reading research articles it is common to see the study hypothesis named the **alternative hypothesis** (alternative to the null hypothesis).

Limitations of clinical trials

The main limitation is budget; clinical trials tend to be expensive to run because it may be necessary to screen multiple animals to find one that has all of the inclusion criteria and none of the exclusion criteria, and it usually becomes expensive to maintain animals under specific circumstances to control the exposure. They usually require excellent records to control all possible risk factors and scenarios that could alter the outcome.

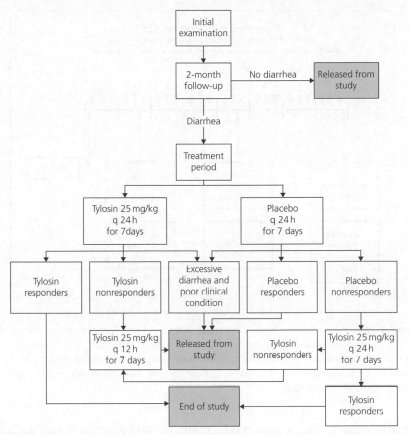

Figure 4.7 Schematic representation of the study design of a clinical trial of the effect of tylosin on diarrhea in dogs (Kilpinen, S., Spillmann, T., Syrja, P., Skrzypczak, T., Louhelainen, M., & Westermarck, E. (2011). Effect of tylosin on dogs with suspected tylosin-responsive diarrhea: a placebo-controlled, randomized, double-blinded, prospective clinical trial. *Acta Veterinaria Scandinavica*, **53**:26).

Advantages of clinical trials

They are the best option to prove causal relationship between a potential risk factor and an outcome.

Sampling strategies

Once we know what type of study we are dealing with, it is important to ensure that the differences in the study groups are due to the effect of the risk factors only and not due to other reasons. The best strategy that allows minimization of differences in characteristics among animals in the different study groups is **random sampling**, where each animal has the same chance to be entered in a study group. This strategy is best implemented using a random generator and

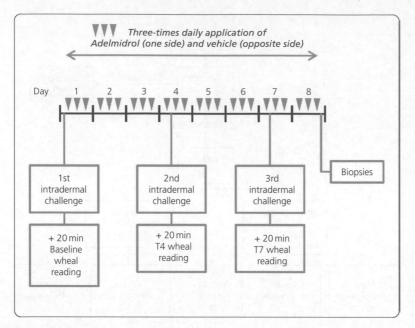

Figure 4.8 Schematic representation of the study design and timeline of a clinical trial of the effect of topical adelmidrol on skin health in dogs (Cerrato, S., Brazis, P., Della Valle, M.F., Miolo, A., & Puigdemont, A. (2012). Inhibitory effect of topical adelmidrol on antigen-induced skin wheal and mast cell behavior in a canine model of allergic dermatitis. *BMC Veterinary Research*, **8**:230–238).

then assigning the next animal to the group identified by the random number. There are free random generators online, and Microsoft Excel® has some functions that build a list of random numbers.

• The simplest random number generator function in Excel is as follows:

$$= \text{RAND}() \tag{4.1}$$

This formula will generate a random number between 0 and 1 with as many decimal points as desired. If the number is formatted to be an integer (i.e., no decimal points), this formula will result in either a value of 0 or 1. This function is useful for studies that involve only two groups.

• The most functional random number generator function in Excel is as follows:

$$= \text{RANDBETWEEN}(x, y) \tag{4.2}$$

where x and y are numbers you identify. The result of this formula is an integer between the two established numbers (x and y). This function is especially useful in studies that involve more than two groups.

Random sampling will allow comparable groups through an equal distribution of commonly evaluated characteristics such as gender, age, and breed among the study groups, as well as other characteristics that are not always known that could bias the result of the study. This is the reason why this strategy is the best suited for clinical trials. However, random sampling is not always feasible in practice. In these cases, there are other sampling strategies that allow minimization of differences between the study groups, although not at the same level as random sampling. Below are some of the most useful and common sampling strategies, but it is important to emphasize that they are not random and they are therefore subject to include some type of bias in a study.

Systematic sampling

This strategy involves enrollment of animals into a study group at equal intervals; most commonly, one animal is enrolled into one group and the next animal presented is enrolled into the other group (if only two study groups). When more than two study groups are involved, each presented animal is enrolled in one group in an organized manner, following always the same order (Group A, Group B, and Group C).

Example

Assume, for example, that a clinical trial wants to compare the effect of iodine or chlorhexidine solution on wound healing using actual canine patients in a veterinary clinic. Dogs could be enrolled alternatingly to use either iodine or chlorhexidine. If the study were to also evaluate peroxide as a third study group, the systematic sampling strategy would require each new dog to be systematically included in the next group, always in the same order: for example, Group A—iodine, Group B—chlorhexidine, and Group C—peroxide.

Systematic sampling also occurs when a study is performed in a horse barn and horses are enrolled by location. For example, the first horse is included in the treated group, the next horse in the control group, the next in the treated group, etc.

A commonly used sampling strategy that is usually miscategorized as random sampling when in fact it is a type of systematic sampling involves the use of some type of number identification that has been assigned to the animal, such as an ear tag number or a microchip number. It is common in these situations to enroll even numbers in one study group and odd numbers in the other study group. Although it may help in reducing bias, it is not a random sampling strategy and it should not be considered as such.

Stratified sampling

This sampling strategy involves enrolment of animals grouping them by certain characteristics that we know could possibly affect the results, typically gender, age, breed, and disposition or use (racing, show, hunting, etc.). Within each stratum, animals can be assigned to the treatment or control group randomly, systematically, or by convenience.

Haphazard or convenient sampling

This strategy involves enrolment of a convenient group of animals in the study groups, such as the first 5 or 10 dogs seen each morning at a clinic because the days get complicated past a certain hour to accurately collect all the information needed. However, these animals most likely have certain characteristics in common that differentiate them from the entire population, such as being owned by retirees that have no other dependents and therefore spend inordinate amount of time, effort, and resources on their pets.

Example

Assume a study of the effect of exercise on obesity in dogs, where the convenience sample is the first five dogs that come into the clinic each morning and each afternoon. Owners in the treatment group are instructed to provide their dogs with an extra 30 min of exercise each day, while owners in the control group are instructed to not alter their habits. If the first five dogs that are seen in the mornings all belong to retirees in their 70s who lead a sedentary life, the 30 min of exercise could be considered as a slow stroll in the park, while the first five dogs in the afternoon could belong to college students who have no classes at that time and decide to bring the dog in for the annual vaccination. The college students may implement the extra 30 min of exercise playing with a Frisbee in the park or taking their dog out on a 3-mile run. It is very likely that this study will result in biased results, probably leaning toward an answer that extra exercise does not help control obesity.

Another example of convenient sampling involves enrollment of wildlife that is presented at rescue facilities because it is easily accessible for biological samples, when in reality these animals are likely not representative of the population because some factor made them more susceptible to be struck by a vehicle on the road or to be easily captured. In farms that have multiple animals in a semi-confinement setting, the first 10 horses or cows to enter from the paddock or pasture into a pen are most likely the dominant animals of the group, while the sick ones are most likely the last ones. Convenient sampling is the least preferred sampling strategy due to the likely presence of one or more possible confounding factors (Chapter 2).

---

5 Causation versus association

Understanding the difference between **causation** and association will be a major keystone for determining which risk factors need to be accounted for and studied more in depth when looking at diseased animals and which risk factors are present fortuitously.

> The example most commonly used to show the difference between causation and association is from the human medicine literature. In 1965, Sir Austin Bradford Hill, professor of medical statistics, outlined the methodic determination of causal risk factors (Hill 1965) using examples from the human literature such as the report from the Advisory Board to the Surgeon General on Smoke and Health. In that report both smoking and drinking showed significant association with lung cancer. However, as we know now, only smoking is a causal risk factor for lung cancer. The reason why drinking showed a positive association with lung cancer was because many people who smoked also drank.
>
> An example from the veterinary literature would be retinal degeneration in cats that were fed dog food (Aguirre 1978). However, other cats that reportedly were consuming dog food were not suffering from retinal degeneration. The causative factor was determined to be taurine deficiency, which is an amino acid not commonly included in commercial dog food; the dog food per se was not the problem. Some commercial dog foods include some minor levels of taurine that along with some table scraps or other sources of food may have been enough to prevent retinal degeneration.

Association is the measurable relationship between two variables (not necessarily risk factor and outcome). Causation is the measureable relationship between a risk factor and the outcome that implies the presence of the risk factor to obtain the outcome. So what are the distinctive features that make a risk factor a causal factor, as opposed to simply a factor associated with the disease or

Practical Clinical Epidemiology for the Veterinarian, First Edition. Aurora Villarroel.
© 2015 John Wiley & Sons, Inc. Published 2015 by John Wiley & Sons, Inc.
Companion website: www.wiley.com/go/villarroel/epidemiology

condition? We will follow the steps provided by the Surgeon General interlaced with examples related to a clever analogy comparing disease causation to criminal law (Evans 1978).

Hill's criteria to determine causation

Temporal association

This is the most important criterion for a risk factor to be considered a causal factor; *a causative risk factor has to be present before the outcome is observed*. A risk factor that is observed only after the intended outcome is diagnosed cannot be established as a cause of the outcome. In the analogy with criminal law, you would not determine a suspect is the criminal if you can only link him to the victim or crime scene after the crime happened, but not before.

> **Example**
>
> Assume a study of incidence of sarcoma in cats during a rabies vaccine campaign of feral cats. Any cat that is diagnosed with a sarcoma at the time of vaccination could not be deemed to be caused by the vaccine because the sarcomas were already present. It does not mean that vaccines cannot be associated with sarcoma in other populations (as we know this happens to be true), it just means that in that specific population, it is not likely because a prior vaccination of a feral cat is unlikely.

It seems silly to dwell on this, but it will make the difference in many situations in which we are trying to establish causal factors for a new condition. It is important to note here that the two most common types of studies used in the veterinary literature, retrospective studies and cross-sectional studies (see Chapter 4), are not suited to establish causality precisely because it may not be possible to establish whether the potential causative factor was in place before the outcome or disease. To establish causality, it is necessary to have non-diseased animals at the beginning of a study and to follow them up over time to determine if and when they develop disease. Otherwise, it would be a case of "which came first, the chicken or the egg."

> Temporal association: a causal risk factor has to be present before the outcome is observed.

Strength of association

To be considered causal, a risk factor needs to be strongly associated with the outcome. A weak association could indicate that the risk factor and the outcome are haphazardly appearing together in some animals. We will learn in the second part of this chapter how to measure the strength of an association.

Consistency of association

The relationship between the risk factor and the outcome needs to be consistent and repeatable over time, in different studies and under different circumstances. As aforementioned, an inconsistent association most likely indicates the potential risk factor and the studied outcome are not really related but appear haphazardly together in some animals. This is why it is important to repeat studies, to seek that consistency. It is not uncommon to find studies with different and even opposing conclusions on the relationship of a potential risk factor and a studied outcome, most likely because there are other factors influencing this relationship (see Chapter 2).

Example

Multiple studies have shown the association between vaccination and development of fibrosarcoma at the injection site. This association seems to be more consistent for rabies and FeLV (feline leukemia virus) vaccines than other vaccines (Kass *et al.* 1993). Because of this consistent association of vaccination sites and tumor development, a task force was established that developed recommendations for specific vaccination sites (Anonymous 1999). The guidelines establish that rabies vaccines are administered in the right rear leg (as distal as possible), FeLV vaccines are administered in the left rear leg (as distal as possible), and other vaccines are administered in the right shoulder, avoiding the midline or interscapular space. These recommendations will allow for two things: (i) identification of the culprit of the tumor and (ii) amputation to save the animal's life in case a tumor develops.

If the association is causal, it should be possible to induce the outcome experimentally by applying the causal risk factor. This is one of the basics of Koch's postulates. Additionally, eliminating the causal risk factor should prevent the outcome or at least reduce it.

Example

Continuing with the sarcoma example, sarcomas should be then preventable by not injecting vaccines. However, there are other causes of sarcomas, so sarcomas will continue to exist even though we can reduce their incidence by not injecting vaccines in cats.

Replication of the study and finding consistent results is the best way to ensure that the identified risk factors are truly associated with the outcome under study.

Specificity of association

The specificity of an association refers to the fact that a risk factor is to be mostly associated with the studied outcome and no other outcomes. It is to be expected that this rule is the most flexible, as we know that some causal factors can result in multiple outcomes.

Example

Parvovirus in dogs can be the cause of diarrhea in puppies and cardiac pathology. In medicine, these are considered as two different syndromes of the same disease, but in epidemiology, they are two different outcomes related to the same causative agent.

Dose–response (biological gradient)

This rule does not apply in all circumstances, but when present, it does identify a risk factor. The dose–response criterion establishes a relationship between the amount of risk factor present and the amount of outcome observed. It could be a direct relationship: increasing amounts of a risk factor increase the amount of the outcome. For example, the more antifreeze a dog ingests, the more damage to its kidneys. It can also be an inverse relationship, where increasing amounts of a risk factor decrease the amount of outcome, or decreasing amounts of risk factor increase the amount of outcome. For example, the higher the insulin dose, the lower the glucose concentration in serum.

Example

For example, in a study of dystocia in Boxers (Linde Forsberg and Persson 2007), the authors reported an increasing frequency of dystocia as the age of the dam increased (Figure 5.1).

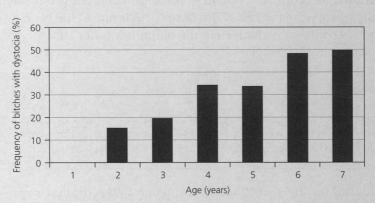

Figure 5.1 Age distribution of 70 whelping Boxers that needed veterinary treatment (Linde Forsberg, F.C. & Persson, G. (2007). A survey of dystocia in the Boxer breed. *Acta Veterinaria Scandinavica*, **49**:8).

An example of an inverse dose–effect is presented in a study of the effect of a recombinant tissue-type plasminogen activator on thrombolysis in horses (Baumer *et al.* 2013). In this study, the authors found that higher doses of the plasminogen activator resulted in ever-decreasing thrombus weight (Figure 5.2).

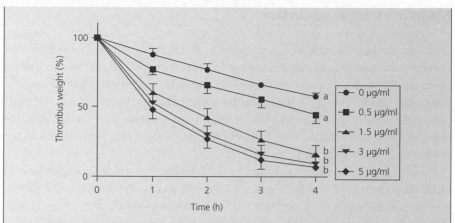

Figure 5.2 Change in risk of vaccine-associated tumors in cats according to the number of vaccines received (Kass, P.H., Barnes, W.G., Jr., Spangler, W.L., Chomel, B.B., & Culbertson, M.R. (1993). Epidemiologic evidence for a causal relation between vaccination and fibrosarcoma tumorigenesis in cats. *Journal of the American Veterinary Medical Association*, **203**:396–405. © AVMA).

Biologic plausibility

The relationship between the causal risk factor and the outcome needs to make biological sense. In the Surgeon General's example about human lung cancer, the association with drinking did not seem plausible, while that with smoking made sense. However, this criterion can be obscured by limitations of the scientific knowledge at the time of the evaluation. Imagine the early times of relatively recently discovered diseases such as bovine spongiform encephalopathy (mad cow disease), West Nile virus infection, or canine influenza.

> Using the criminal law analogy by Evans, the criminal should have a motive.

Analogy

Similar diseases in different populations have similar associations to a causal risk factor. This is in fact how we initially evaluate most causal risk factors; in other words, "do we know of a similar condition in another species?" For example, at the beginning of the outbreak of canine influenza, it was not known that the cause was a virus. However, there were multiple analogies to human influenza cases, and this led to the discovery of the canine influenza virus.

> **Example**
>
> In 2010, a horse in Australia was diagnosed with fibrosarcoma at the injection site of the equine influenza vaccine 6 months earlier. Although fibrosarcoma in horses due to vaccine reactions is not a common occurrence, the vaccine was deemed as the causative agent in this case given the similarity with the vaccine-associated sarcomas in cats. Although this is a single case example (not in a population), it may eventually become a more common diagnosis once the potential risk factor is recognized in horses.

Measures of association

There are several measures of association that can be used in epidemiology, but knowing the main measures reported in the literature will enable you to understand studies and help you to interpret their results, so you can apply them into your daily work. There are two main measures used in the literature, the odds ratio (OR) and the relative risk (RR). Additionally, we will cover the attributable risk (AR) due to its importance in establishing the most likely associated factor in outbreak investigations (Chapter 7).

This is one place where the famous 2×2 tables that epidemiologists use so often come into play (Table 5.1). A 2×2 table is a cross-tabulation of variables. The most common way to organize the 2×2 table is using the outcome variable as the column variable and the risk factor under study as the row variable. where

- a is the number of animals that were exposed to that risk factor and became diseased,
- b is the number of animals that were exposed and did not become diseased,
- c is the number of animals that were not exposed and became diseased, and
- d is the number of animals that were not exposed and did not become diseased.

To not get confused with "yes" and "no" on both the columns and the rows, it is best to set the table up as diseased (Dz) and nondiseased (No-Dz) or affected and nonaffected (Table 5.2). You can choose any terminology you prefer, but we suggest choosing something different than "+" and "−" because this is usually the terminology used for results of diagnostic tests (see Chapter 6).

Table 5.1 Organization of a 2×2 table for analysis of risk factors.

		Disease status		
		Yes	No	
Risk factor	Yes	a	b	$a+b$
	No	c	d	$c+d$
		$a+c$	$b+d$	Total

Table 5.2 Simplified layout of a 2×2 table for analysis of risk factors.

		Dz	No-Dz	
Risk factor	Yes	a	b	$a+b$
	No	b	d	$c+d$
		$a+c$	$b+d$	Total

Once you have this setup clear, you can test anything as a risk factor. The important thing is to remember that all animals in the population under study have to be included in the table, as part of either the exposed group or the unexposed group.

Example

To test the association of pasture access (risk factor) with a possible development of musculoskeletal injuries (outcome or disease), the setup of the 2×2 table would be as exposed in Table 5.3.

Table 5.3 Organization of the 2×2 table for analysis of exposure to pasture as a risk factor for injuries in horses.

		Injury	OK	
Risk factor	Pasture	a	b	a+b
	No pasture	c	d	c+d
		a+c	b+d	Total

Another way of coding this 2×2 table would be as in Table 5.4.

Table 5.4 Organization of the 2×2 table for analysis of exposure to pasture as a risk factor for injuries in horses (alternative coding).

		Injury	OK	
Pasture	Yes	a	b	a+b
	No	c	d	c+d
		a+c	b+d	Total

This way the risk factor is easily identified at the leftmost part of the table, and every 2×2 table would look similar (yes/no for the risk factor) making it easier to follow.

To test the association of having more than one pet (risk factor) with behavioral problems in dogs (outcome), the 2×2 table would be set up as in Table 5.5.

Another way of coding this 2×2 table would be as in Table 5.6.

Table 5.5 Organization of the 2×2 table for analysis of exposure to multiple pets as a risk factor for behavioral problems in dogs.

		Abnormal	Normal	
Risk factor	Multiple pets	a	b	a+b
	Single pet	c	d	c+d
		a+c	b+d	Total

Table 5.6 Organization of the 2×2 table for analysis of exposure to multiple pets as a risk factor for behavioral problems in dogs (alternative coding).

		Abnormal	Normal	
Multiple pets	Yes	a	b	a+b
	No	c	d	c+d
		a+c	b+d	Total

Table 5.7 Visualization of the calculation of the odds ratio.

		Disease status Yes	Disease status No
Risk factor	Yes	a	b
	No	c	d

A clear setup of the 2×2 table will allow evaluation of anything as a risk factor.

Odds ratio

The OR is defined as the odds of disease in exposed versus nonexposed animals. It is a ratio of ratios, which can also be called ratio of odds because remember that an odd is a ratio.

The formula for the OR is derived as follows:

$$\text{OR} = \frac{\text{Odds of disease in exposed animals}}{\text{Odds of disease in nonexposed animals}} = \frac{a/c}{b/d} = \frac{a \cdot d}{b \cdot c} \quad (5.1)$$

Notice that this formula can be easily seen as multiplying across diagonals and dividing one diagonal by the other (Table 5.7).

The important part of this is how to interpret the result. In other words, what does OR=X mean?

Interpretation: The odds to develop disease are X times greater in exposed animals than in nonexposed animals.

Example

Assume we want to study the effect of racing as a risk factor for developing lameness in horses. We have a population of 100 horses, half of them are racing (risk factor) and the other half do not race. We observe that 30 of the racing horses develop lameness, while only five of the nonracing horses are lame.

First, we set up the 2×2 table with the information we have (Table 5.8).

Table 5.8 Setup of the 2×2 table with information from a study on lame horses.

		Lame	OK	
Racing	Yes	30	—	50
	No	5	—	50
		—	—	100

The rest of the table can be calculated from the data we have. Calculations are shown in parentheses in each cell. The complete table would look like Table 5.9.

Table 5.9 Calculation of empty cells in a 2×2 table based on existing data on lame horses.

		Lame	OK	
Racing	Yes	30	$(50-30)=20$	50
	No	5	$(50-5)=45$	50
		$(30+5)=35$	$(20+45)=$ $(100-35)=65$	100

$$OR = \frac{a \cdot d}{b \cdot c} = \frac{30 \cdot 45}{20 \cdot 5} = \frac{1350}{100} = 13.5 \qquad (5.2)$$

Interpretation: Horses that race are (according to this example) 13.5 times more likely to develop lameness than nonracing horses.

Because the OR is a ratio, it can acquire values between 0 and infinity. So what does each value mean?

- *OR = 1* means both groups (exposed and nonexposed) are equally likely to develop the disease or condition of study.
- *OR > 1* implies a *positive association* between the studied variable and the disease, meaning that it is more likely for an exposed animal to have the disease than a nonexposed animal; the studied variable is a risk factor.
- *OR < 1* implies a *negative association*, meaning that an exposed animal is more likely to *not develop the disease* (be healthy) than a nonexposed animal; the studied variable is *protective* or *preventive*.

Side note: Often, we hear the term "preventative" instead of the correct form preventive. Although it is not known how this term came into usage, it is common to hear people use similar words with more syllables to sound more erudite (such as saying "utilizing" instead of "using"). Over time, it has become a commonly used term and has been accepted in the dictionary as an alternative form of the correct term, but using "preventative" is grammatically incorrect given that the verb is "to prevent," not "to preventate." So, after reading this, please, do not ever use the wrong term again.

This last scenario is seen typically when evaluating the effect of vaccination on developing a disease when the "exposed" group (first row in the 2×2 table) is defined as the vaccinated group.

Example

In studying the effect of vaccination as a *protective factor* against developing feline leukemia infection in cats (Hines *et al.* 1991), we have the following table presented (Figure 5.3).

Vaccine No.*	Persistent viremia (No./total)		No. of transiently viremic vaccinates
	Vaccinates	Controls	
1	0/16	4/4	0/16
2	0/11	4/4	1/11
3	1/10	5/5	1/9
4 and 5	2/13	4/5	0/11
6	1/6	4/5	1/5
7 (IM)†	2/44	16/22	3/42
7 (SC)†	6/44	...	4/38
Total	12/144 (8%)	39/45 (87%)	10/132 (6%)

*Each number was a separately prepared vaccine
†Route of vaccine administration.

Figure 5.3 Comparison of viremia observed in cats vaccinated against feline leukemia and control cats (Hines, D.L., Cutting, J.A., Dietrich, D.L., & Walsh, J.A. (1991). Evaluation of efficacy and safety of an inactivated virus vaccine against feline leukemia virus infection. *Journal of the American Veterinary Medical Association*, **199**:1428–1430. © AVMA).

Concentrate on the overall results of the table, presented in the last row (Total). We have 144 vaccinated cats and 45 control cats. We set up the 2×2 table with the information we have (Table 5.10).

Table 5.10 Setup of the 2×2 table with information from a study on viremia in cats vaccinated against feline leukemia.

		Viremia	OK	
Vaccinated	Yes	12		144
	No	39		45

The rest of the table can be calculated (Table 5.11) from the data we have (calculations are shown in parentheses within each cell).

Table 5.11 Calculation of empty cells in a 2×2 table based on existing data on viremia in cats vaccinated against feline leukemia.

		Viremia	OK	
Vaccinated	Yes	12	$(144 - 12) = 132$	144
	No	39	$(45 - 39) = 6$	45
		$(12 + 39) = 51$	$\begin{matrix}(132 + 6) = \\ (189 - 51) =\end{matrix} 138$	189

$$\text{OR} = \frac{a \cdot d}{b \cdot c} = \frac{12 \cdot 6}{132 \cdot 39} = \frac{72}{5148} = 0.014 \tag{5.3}$$

Interpretation: Vaccinated cats are (according to this example) 0.014 times LESS likely to develop viremia than nonvaccinated cats.

When a risk factor shows an $\text{OR} < 1$, it is called a **protective risk factor**. However, it is usually difficult to visualize, and therefore it is commonly "translated" to be presented in the light of a positive association. This can be achieved by inverting the result (1/OR) or by inverting the risk factor in the 2×2 table so that the "exposed" animals are those not vaccinated.

Following with the aforementioned example, if the OR = 0.014 is inverted, the resulting OR is:

$$\frac{1}{0.014} = 71.5 \tag{5.4}$$

The **interpretation** now would be that "nonvaccinated" cats are 71.5 times MORE likely to develop viremia than vaccinated cats.

Let us invert the 2×2 table and go through the calculations to prove that the result is the same (Table 5.12).

Table 5.12 Setup of the 2×2 table with information from a study on viremia in cats vaccinated against feline leukemia, assuming that vaccination against feline leukemia is protective.

		Viremia	OK	
Vaccinated	No	39	$(45 - 39) = 6$	45
	Yes	12	$(144 - 12) = 132$	144
		$(12 + 39) = 51$	$\begin{matrix}(132 + 6) = \\ (189 - 51) =\end{matrix} 138$	189

$$\text{OR} = \frac{a \cdot d}{b \cdot c} = \frac{39 \cdot 132}{6 \cdot 12} = \frac{5148}{72} = 71.5 \tag{5.5}$$

Interpretation: Nonvaccinated cats are (according to this example) 71.5 times more likely to develop viremia than vaccinated cats.

Another way of looking at this when setting up the inverted 2×2 table is assuming that nonvaccinated animals are more vulnerable to the disease agent than vaccinated animals. This way, if the vaccine is protective (as expected), the OR will be larger than 1 and will be easier to interpret. Notice however that vaccination can be a risk factor for another condition while being protective for the disease it was designed.

Example

In the examples presented previously on the development of fibrosarcoma at vaccination sites in cats, if we were to study the effect of vaccination on developing localized cancer, we would set up the 2×2 table (Table 5.13) using vaccination as the exposure factor (first row).

Table 5.13 Organization of the 2×2 table for evaluation of vaccination against feline leukemia as a risk factor for fibrosarcoma in cats.

		Fibrosarcoma	OK
Vaccinated	Yes	a	c
	No	b	d

Using data from the study by Kass *et al.* in 1993, information about the association of fibrosarcoma development with the injection of various vaccines is presented in one of the tables in the paper (Figure 5.4).

Vaccine	Cases			Controls			OR	95% CI
	EXP	Not EXP	Unknown	EXP	Not EXP	Unknown		
FeLV[*]	41	41	22	36	102	37	2.82	1.54 to 5.15
FVRCP[*]	50	41	13	66	75	34	1.40	0.80 to 2.43
Pneumonitis-chlamydia[*]	6	66	32	16	103	56	0.54	0.19 to 1.49
Rabies[*]	22	70	12	20	118	37	2.09	1.01 to 4.31
Rabies[†]	7	26	8	17	106	37	1.83	0.65 to 5.10

[*]Case fibrosarcomas in cervical/interscapular region; EXP indicates vaccination in cervical/interscapular region.
[†] Case fibrosarcomes in femoral region; EXP indicates vaccination in femoral region.
EXP = exposed to vaccination at tumor site; CI = confidence interval.

Figure 5.4 Comparison of tumors observed in vaccination sites versus other locations in cats (Kass, P.H., Barnes, W.G., Jr., Spangler, W.L., Chomel, B.B., & Culbertson, M.R. (1993). Epidemiologic evidence for a causal relation between vaccination and fibrosarcoma tumorigenesis in cats. *Journal of the American Veterinary Medical Association*, **203**:396–405. © AVMA).

The first line shows the association with FeLV vaccination. Let us build the 2×2 table (Table 5.14).

Table 5.14 Setup of the 2×2 table with information from a study on vaccine-associated tumor in cats vaccinated against feline leukemia.

		Fibrosarcoma (cases)	OK (controls)
Vaccinated	Yes (*exposed*)	41	36
	No (*not exposed*)	41	102

Those cats with unknown exposure are not included in the analyses. Now we calculate the OR:

$$OR = \frac{a \cdot d}{b \cdot c} = \frac{41 \cdot 102}{36 \cdot 41} = \frac{4182}{1476} = 2.83 \qquad (5.6)$$

You can observe that the resulting OR is very close to the one listed on the first line in the table of the published article. The reason for not being exactly the same is most likely rounding due to decimal points. The interpretation of this OR is that cats vaccinated with FeLV were 2.82 times more likely to develop fibrosarcoma than nonvaccinated cats.

Comparing the OR of all other vaccines, it is evident that not all vaccines were associated with fibrosarcoma development in that study. For interpretation of the 95% confidence interval, please see the section "Confidence interval" in Chapter 2.

The OR can be used in prospective and retrospective studies and is thus the most common measure of association used in the veterinary literature.

Relative risk

RR is defined as the risk (probability) of exposed animals to develop disease versus the risk of nonexposed animals to develop disease. In other words, how much more likely is an animal to develop disease when exposed to the study variable than when not exposed. It is a proportion of proportions.

The formula for the risk of exposed animals to develop disease is:

$$\text{Risk}_{\text{exposed}} = \frac{a}{a+b} \qquad (5.7)$$

The formula for the risk of nonexposed animals to develop disease is:

$$\text{Risk}_{\text{nonexposed}} = \frac{c}{c+d} \qquad (5.8)$$

The RR is calculated by dividing one risk by the other:

$$RR = \frac{\text{Risk that an exposed animal develops disease}}{\text{Risk that a nonexposed animal develops disease}} = \frac{\text{Risk}_{\text{exposed}}}{\text{Risk}_{\text{nonexposed}}} = \frac{\frac{a}{a+b}}{\frac{c}{c+d}}$$

$$(5.9)$$

The most common study designs evaluated with the RR are field trials, in which two separate groups of animals are included in the study, one exposed to the study variable and one not exposed. Then the risk of disease is calculated in exposed and nonexposed individuals. Note that these are prospective studies. Another common example is the use in cross-sectional studies.

Example

Consider the table in Figure 5.5 obtained from a study that evaluated the effect of several potential risk factors on the development of mammary cancer in dogs (Schneider *et al.* 1969). This table presents data on the number of estrous cycles the dogs had before spaying as a risk factor for developing mammary tumors. We will use the term "sexually immature" to identify dogs that had never exhibited an estrous cycle before spaying. Dogs showing one or more estrous cycles are lumped together for analysis.

Number of estrous cycles before neutering*	Number of mammary cases		Number of controls observed	$x^{2\dagger}$	Relative risk†
	Observed	Expected†			
None	1	15.05	26	37.26	0.005
1	3	9.34	11	12.85	0.08
2 or more	20	28.69	25	10.06	0.26

* Not neutered: 63 cases, 23 controls: neutered at an unknown age: 2 controls.
† The expected number, χ^2 (df = 1), and relative risk were computed by the Mantel-Haenszel procedure, with age controlled and effect of various numbers of estrous cycles before neutering tested separately for each group, against bitches never neutered; $\chi^2 \geq 3.84$ is statistically significant at the 5% level or less.

Figure 5.5 Effects of sexual maturity (number of estrous cycles) prior to spaying on the risk of developing mammary cancer in dogs (Schneider, R., Dorn, C.R., & Taylor, D.O. (1969). Factors influencing canine mammary cancer development and postsurgical survival. *Journal of the National Cancer Institute*, **43**:1249–1261).

As we did before, we fill the 2 × 2 table with the data we have (Table 5.15).

Table 5.15 Setup of the 2 × 2 table with information from a study on the effect of spaying on the development of mammary cancer in dogs.

		Cancer (cases)	OK (controls)
Sexually immature	Yes (*exposed*)	1	26
	No (*not exposed*)	(3 + 20) = 23	(11 + 25) = 36

Now we calculate the missing cells (Table 5.16).

Table 5.16 Calculation of empty cells in a 2×2 table based on existing data on the effect of spaying on the development of mammary cancer in dogs.

		Cancer (cases)	OK (controls)	
Sexually immature	Yes (*exposed*)	1	26	$(1+26)=27$
	No (*not exposed*)	23	36	$(23+36)=59$
		$(1+23)=24$	$(26+36)=62$	86

$$RR = \frac{Risk_{exposed}}{Risk_{nonexposed}} = \frac{\dfrac{a}{a+b}}{\dfrac{c}{c+d}} = \frac{\dfrac{1}{1+26}}{\dfrac{23}{23+36}} = \frac{\dfrac{1}{27}}{\dfrac{23}{59}} = \frac{0.04}{0.39} = 0.10 \tag{5.10}$$

Interpretation: Dogs that were spayed while sexually immature were 0.10 times at less risk to develop mammary cancer than dogs that were sexually mature. In this case, we can see spaying early is a protective factor against mammary cancer in dogs.

As we saw with the OR, an $RR < 1$ is considered a protective factor, while an $RR > 1$ is considered a risk factor. We could set up the 2×2 table in the inverse order (Table 5.17) if we expect the study factor to be protective, as would likely happen with a supplement product, a vaccine, or some interventions.

Table 5.17 Alternate setup of the 2×2 table with information from a study on the effect of spaying on the development of mammary cancer in dogs.

		Cancer (cases)	OK (controls)
Sexually immature	No (*exposed*)	23	36
	Yes (*not exposed*)	1	26

Sometimes, it is more intuitive to change the name of the exposure to be the opposite of the protective factor, so it becomes more obvious what the risk factor is.

For the example at hand, instead of using "sexually immature" as the risk factor under study (as it has proven to be protective), we could set up the 2×2 table using "sexually mature" or "previous estrus" as the exposure variable to make interpretation clearer. This way we keep the exposed and nonexposed animals in the top and bottom row of the 2×2 table, making it easier to follow (Table 5.18).

Table 5.18 Alternate naming of the exposure variable in the 2×2 table with information from a study on the effect of spaying on the development of mammary cancer in dogs.

		Cancer (cases)	OK (controls)
Sexually mature	Yes (*exposed*)	23	36
(previous estrus)	No (*not exposed*)	1	26

Now, we calculate the RR:

$$RR = \frac{Risk_{exposed}}{Risk_{nonexposed}} = \frac{\dfrac{a}{a+b}}{\dfrac{c}{c+d}} = \frac{\dfrac{23}{23+36}}{\dfrac{1}{1+26}} = \frac{\dfrac{23}{59}}{\dfrac{1}{27}} = \frac{0.39}{0.04} = 9.75 \qquad (5.11)$$

Interpretation: Dogs spayed after reaching sexual maturity (indicated by at least one estrous cycle) are 9.75 times more likely to develop mammary cancer than dogs spayed while sexually immature.

The RR can be used only in prospective studies as it looks at the risk of disease given that an animal is exposed or not. It is not that common to see RR in the veterinary literature anymore, but it is important to present as the comparison for the OR.

It may be confusing to differentiate well between odds and risk of developing disease.

- **Risk** is the probability of an event happening in the present or the future within a population. It is a proportion and, therefore, the numerator is included in the denominator in the formula.
- **Odds**, being a ratio, compares the likelihood of an event happening in two mutually exclusive groups: the numerator is not included in the denominator. Odds may indicate either a future or a past association.

Taking into account these differences, it becomes evident that the RR can only be used to evaluate prospective studies (see Chapter 4), while the OR can be used for any study. This is why it is so important to understand the interpretation of the OR as it is the most widely used measure of association used in the medical literature.

OR can be used to evaluate any study, RR only in prospective studies.

Attributable risk

The AR measures the absolute difference between the risk of an exposed animal to develop disease and the risk of a nonexposed animal to develop disease. In other words, it measures the difference in risk of disease associated with the presence of the study variable, taking into account that there is a certain risk of disease that is due to other risk factors that are already present in the population. The reason to use the absolute value of the difference is that when a protective factor is considered the exposure variable, the difference would be negative. When considering the risk that is attributable to a factor, it should have no sign (positive or negative).

It is calculated as a simple difference in absolute values between the risk of disease in exposed animals and that in nonexposed animals. The risk of disease in nonexposed animals is considered the baseline of disease in the population.

The formula to calculate the AR is:

$$AR = Risk_{exposed} - Risk_{nonexposed} \tag{5.12}$$

Notice that these are the same terms used in RR, but they are subtracted as opposed to divided.

Example

Using the example we used for the RR, the AR for mammary cancer due to sexual maturity is:

$$AR = \left(Risk_{exposed} - Risk_{nonexposed}\right) = \left(\frac{23}{59} - \frac{1}{27}\right) = 0.39 - 0.04 = 0.35 \tag{5.13}$$

Interpretation: The delay in spaying after achieving sexual maturity accounts for 35% of the risk of mammary cancer in the study population.

This measurement will prove very valuable when investigating outbreaks (Chapter 7).

6   Diagnostic tests

Most people consider a diagnostic test to be some device that analyzes a fluid or tissue sample and provides a reading (numeric or colorimetric). However, these types of diagnostic tests represent only a small part of all the diagnostic tests used in daily practice. The word "diagnosis" comes from two Greek words: "dia" (apart) and "gignoskein" (to recognize or know). In essence, diagnosis means the ability to differentiate or to tell apart. Therefore, a diagnostic test is any device or procedure that has the ability to differentiate a diseased individual from a nondiseased individual.

From the first moment we see a patient, we intuitively start making diagnoses in the sense of differentiating whether the animal presents signs that are consistent with a healthy status or not. Most of these differentiations are done in terms of dichotomies such as bright/dull, alert/depressed, and responsive/nonresponsive, although categories are also common such as for body condition score, lameness score, etc. Unconsciously, most people disregard their main and initial "diagnostic test," visual appraisal of the patient, as nothing more than getting to know the animal.

Past the initial visual exam of the animal, the TPR we all have been taught to start with on any animal exam is one of our main diagnostic tests. The thermometer is a diagnostic test that provides a reading of the internal body temperature of the animal in degrees Fahrenheit or Celsius (continuous variable), which is usually dichotomized as fever/no fever (categorical variable). Using the stethoscope, we evaluate the presence/absence of abnormal sounds or rhythms. After this we may palpate or manipulate certain parts of the animal to determine whether they conform to normal or there is something wrong. Therefore, every day we are performing multiple diagnostic tests that do not require switching an electronic apparatus on.

Practical Clinical Epidemiology for the Veterinarian, First Edition. Aurora Villarroel.
© 2015 John Wiley & Sons, Inc. Published 2015 by John Wiley & Sons, Inc.
Companion website: www.wiley.com/go/villarroel/epidemiology

Having defined what a diagnostic test is, we need to understand the possible shortcomings, so we can determine what we are going to do with the results.

For example, we know that not all sick animals have fever. Even when an animal has an infectious disease, that animal may not develop a fever, either because it may be at an early stage of the disease or it may be moribund so that its body temperature is actually lower than normal. Therefore, if we were to use fever as an absolute must for an animal to be considered infected, we may misdiagnose the prevalence of infection.

The take-home message is that diagnostic tests are not perfect; they have specific weaknesses that need to be understood so that the results of the test can be used appropriately for clinical reasoning. The following parameters of test quality and performance can be used in practice to guide our clinical assessment.

Diagnostic tests are not perfect.

Test quality

The quality of a test refers to its ability to produce precise and accurate results, avoiding measurement errors. Measurement errors are an important limitation of many diagnostic tests. They can be due to the measurement device itself, the operator, or both.

Accuracy
Accuracy is the ability of a test to detect the actual (real) value. Accuracy can be improved by calibrating the apparatus or the operator.

Precision
Precision is the ability of a test to perform consistently when testing the same sample several times. Precision can be improved by taking multiple measurements of the same sample and using the average of the measurements as the result (notice this results in a single average measurement, the multiple measurements cannot be used as independent samples—see Chapter 2, section "Appropriate statistical analyses for multiple samples taken from the same animal").

A common way to represent accuracy and precision is using targets (Figure 6.1). Accuracy determines how many of the shots actually hit the target, while precision determines how close all of the shots are to each other (even if they are off-target).

A test that is precise but not accurate will be "biased" by a similar amount each time it measures (for a review on bias, see Chapter 2).

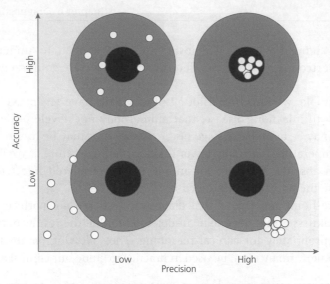

Figure 6.1 Graphical representation of accuracy and precision of a diagnostic test.

Example

Consider the following chemistry panel obtained from a 13-year-old intact male dog (Figure 6.2):

Complete chemistry profile

Animal/Source	Specimen	Specimen type	Date resulted
Hael		Serum	05-Dec-2012

Analyte	Result	Units	Reference interval	Relative result indicator
BUN	23	mg/dL	10–30	
Creatinine	0.8	mg/dL	1.0–2.0	
Glucose	98	mg/dL	65–130	
Cholesterol	217	mg/dL	150–275	
Total Protein	6.8	g/dL	5.4–7.6	
Albumin	3.7	g/dL	2.3–4.0	
Bilirubin, Total	0.2	mg/dL	0.0–0.5	
CK	114	U/L	50–300	
Alkaline Phosphatase	367	U/L	10–84	
GGT	3	U/L	2–10	
ALT (SGPT)	68	U/L	5–65	

Figure 6.2 Partial chemistry panel of a 13-year-old intact male dog.

Looking at the graphical representation of the results, we notice that creatinine is low, while alkaline phosphatase (ALP) and alanine aminotranferase (ALT) are high. At first glance, this panel is consistent with liver disease. However, a closer look at the actual numbers shows that the creatinine and the ALT concentrations are in fact very close to the normal limits. Could the numbers indeed be a problem of precision of the test? In other words, is the creatinine of 0.8 mg/dl really 0.8 and not 0.9 or even 1.0, in which case it would be normal? To answer this question, we would need to know the detection limits for each test (asking the laboratory). A common detection limit for creatinine tests is 0.1 mg/dl, so the reported value of 0.8 mg/dl could in fact be anywhere between 0.7 and 0.9 mg/dl.

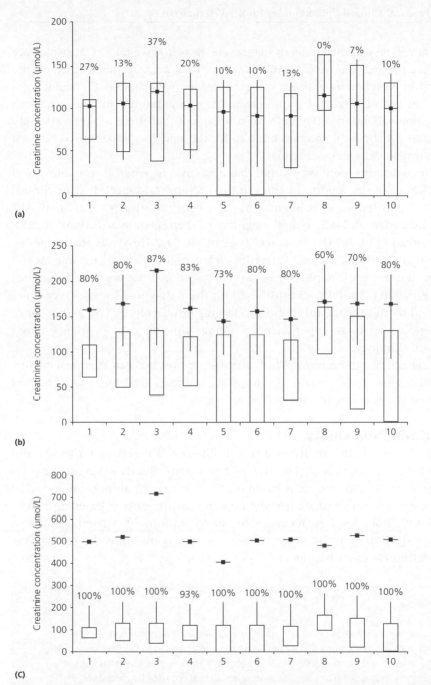

Median creatinine concentrations (μmol/L) and ranges in 10 healthy dogs, 10 dogs with expected intermediate creatinine values and 10 azotemic dogs, analyzed 3 times in different batches by 10 European laboratories (1–10). The horizontal line represent the median. The white background box indicates the reference interval in healthy dogs as specified by each laboratory. Dark grey columns overlaid the upper reference limit, and figures given above them, represent the percentage of dogs that are considered abnormal by use of the upper reference limit for that laboratory. The light grey columns represent the percentage of dogs that are classified as normal. A: 10 healthy dogs, B: 10 dogs with expected intermediate values and C: 10 azotemic dogs.

Figure 6.3 Results of a study on variability of laboratory results on serum creatinine concentrations in dogs (Ulleberg, T., Robben, J., Nordahl, K.M., Ulleberg, T., & Heiene, R. (2011). Plasma creatinine in dogs: intra- and inter-laboratory variation in 10 European veterinary laboratories. *Acta Veterinaria Scandinavica*, **53**:25–53).

You will be surprised to learn that several tests that we take at face value are not very precise, and we continuously make treatment decisions based on the clinical interpretations of those values. Consider, for example, the results of a study on the variability of serum creatinine concentrations in dogs measured in multiple laboratories (Figure 6.3). It is evident that there is large variability of results for the same samples but also for the reference ranges used by each laboratory to determine azotemia.

The next question we would have to ask is what is the biological significance of the reported values in the presence/absence of other clinical signs? Presented in a different way is a concentration of 68 U/l of ALT (normal range of 5–65) equally significant, better, or worse than an ALP concentration of 367 U/l (normal range of 10–84)? How was the range for normal animals established? What does a few points out of the range mean? Given that no test is perfect, these are all questions that we need to ponder before making clinical decisions based on these diagnostic tests. Over time, you will learn to make these interpretations intuitively, as you gather more and more personal experience to guide you in your evidence-based decision-making.

Diagnostic tests are not perfect. There are many factors that can affect test quality, including some problems with the diagnostic test itself and other factors such as operator errors and environmental influence.

Discrimination ability

Discrimination is the ability of a test to differentiate between affected and nonaffected animals. A perfect test will be able to clearly differentiate both states. When the difference is based on the presence or absence of a specific characteristic, it is an easier feat than when the difference is based on reaching a threshold level (a measurable concentration) of a compound in a biological sample. In the latter instance, a "cut-point" must be part of our case definition (see Chapter 1).

Example

Assume we are interested in canine adenovirus exposure. The presence or absence of antibodies will indicate whether or not a dog has been exposed to the virus. However, if our interest is in canine adenovirus infection, we now need to know what level of antibodies is considered an infection as opposed to that provided by vaccination. This is where some tests have better **discrimination ability** than others.

In the graphs in Figure 6.4, the test on the top would be a test with good discrimination ability; infected animals (solid line) have clearly distinguishable antibody titers from noninfected animals. However, in real life, it is much more common to find the situation on the bottom, where some titers such as 1:32 are presented by both infected and noninfected animals. In this situation, an animal presenting a titer of 1:32 would be considered a suspect, and further tests or time would be needed to determine if the animal is infected or not.

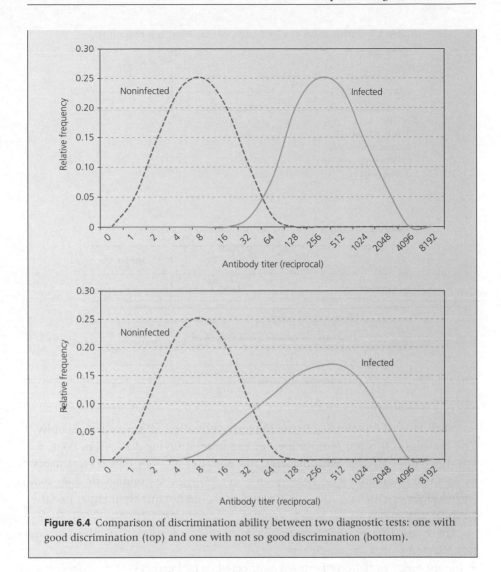

Figure 6.4 Comparison of discrimination ability between two diagnostic tests: one with good discrimination (top) and one with not so good discrimination (bottom).

This is a common problem you will face in your daily practice, and you need to understand what the term "suspect" means and what to do about it. The consequences of misclassifying a "suspect" are different for the animal owner than for the regulatory agency, and you should consider both perspectives.

Test performance

Another important test characteristic is the ability to discriminate between affected and nonaffected (healthy) animals without any ambiguous values (usually labeled as "suspect").

Table 6.1 Organization of a 2 × 2 table for diagnostic test evaluation.

		Dz	No-Dz
Diagnostic test	+	a	b
	−	c	d

where
a, true positive (TP)
b, false positive (FP)
c, false negative (FN)
d, true negative (TN)

Table 6.2 Visualization of test results within a 2 × 2 table.

		Dz	No-Dz
Diagnostic test	+	TP	
	−		TN

		Dz	No-Dz
Diagnostic test	+		FP
	−	FN	

Notice that it is preferable to use the term "nonaffected" instead of "healthy." The reason for this is that if we are, for example, studying diabetes in dogs, we will have dogs affected with diabetes and nonaffected dogs that do not necessarily need to be otherwise healthy. In other words, the nondiabetic dogs may have kidney disease or orthopedic issues that would not qualify them as healthy, so this terminology would be a misnomer.

There are two possible errors in classification of animals as affected and nonaffected with a diagnostic test:
- Identifying a nonaffected animal as affected (type I error)
- Identifying an affected animal as nonaffected (type II error)

The likelihood of a diagnostic test to incur into these errors is given by the specificity and the sensitivity of the test, respectively. The best way to correctly understand these is by classifying the test result using a 2 × 2 table. For the evaluation of diagnostic test performance, the most common way to organize the 2 × 2 table is using the true disease status as the column variable and the diagnostic test results as the row variable (Tables 6.1 and 6.2).

Sensitivity

Sensitivity (Se) is the ability of a test to correctly diagnose affected animals, in other words, the ability to detect truly positive animals. The formula to calculate the sensitivity of a test is the proportion of diseased individuals (denominator) that is positive to the diagnostic test (numerator). Notice that the formula looks only at the left column of the 2×2 table (highlighted in Table 6.3); it concentrates only on affected individuals.

$$\text{Se} = \frac{\text{True positives}}{\text{All affected}} = \frac{\text{TP}}{\text{TP} + \text{FN}} = \frac{a}{a+c} \tag{6.1}$$

Table 6.3 Visualization of cells included in the calculation of **sensitivity** of a diagnostic test in a 2×2 table.

		Dz	No-Dz
Diagnostic test	+	TP	
	−	FN	

Example

A recent paper reported test performance of a new rapid test for rabies in dog saliva (Kasempimolporn *et al.* 2011). Table 1 of this paper reports actual numbers and is presented here (Figure 6.5)

	FAT (brain smears)		PCR (saliva)	
Strip test	+	−	+	−
+	53[*]	10	53	10
−	4	170	4	170
Total	57	180	57	180

FAT = fluorecent antibody test; PCR = polymerase chain reaction;
+ = positive; − = negative
[*] Number of saliva samples.

Figure 6.5 Identification of data needed to calculate the **sensitivity** of a new rapid test developed for the diagnosis of rabies in dog saliva (Kasempimolporn, S., Saengseesom, W., Huadsakul, S., Boonchang, S., & Sitprija, V. (2011). Evaluation of a rapid immunochromatographic test strip for detection of rabies virus in dog saliva samples. *Journal of Veterinary Diagnostic Investigation*, **23**(6):1197–1201. © Sage).

Given that both the brain smears and the saliva PCR had the same results, we will focus only on the saliva PCR, to compare apples with apples (saliva PCR vs. saliva rapid strip test). The true status of the disease is hereby given by the saliva PCR (columns), and the new diagnostic test is represented in the rows. Therefore, the table is already reporting the data in the appropriate format of the 2×2 table, and there is no need to redo it.

$$\text{Se} = \frac{\text{True positives}}{\text{All affected}} = \frac{\text{TP}}{\text{TP} + \text{FN}} = \frac{53}{53+4} = \frac{53}{57} = 93.0\% \tag{6.2}$$

This means that approximately 7 out of every 100 dogs that have rabies are missed by this test. What is the biological significance of this value to you? Is this an acceptable risk you are willing to take?

Specificity

Specificity (Sp) is the ability of a test to correctly diagnose nonaffected animals, in other words, the ability to detect truly negative animals.

The formula to calculate the specificity of a test is the proportion of nonaffected animals (denominator) that is negative to the diagnostic test (numerator). Notice that the formula looks only at the right column of the 2×2 table (highlighted in Table 6.4); it concentrates only on nonaffected individuals.

$$\text{Sp} = \frac{\text{True negatives}}{\text{All nonaffected}} = \frac{\text{TN}}{\text{TN} + \text{FP}} = \frac{d}{d+b} \qquad (6.3)$$

Table 6.4 Visualization of cells included in the calculation of **specificity** of a diagnostic test in a 2×2 table.

		Dz	No-Dz
Diagnostic test	+		FP
	−		TN

Example

Continuing with the rapid saliva strip test for rabies used before (Kasempimolporn *et al.* 2011), we can calculate the specificity of this new test (Figure 6.6).

Strip test	FAT (brain smears) +	−	PCR (saliva) +	−
+	53[*]	10	53	10
−	4	170	4	170
Total	57	180	57	180

FAT = fluorescent antibody test; PCR = polymerase chain reaction; + = positive; − = negative
[*] Number of saliva samples.

Figure 6.6 Identification of data needed to calculate the **specificity** of a new rapid test developed for the diagnosis of rabies in dog saliva (Kasempimolporn, S., Saengseesom, W., Huadsakul, S., Boonchang, S., & Sitprija, V. (2011). Evaluation of a rapid immunochromatographic test strip for detection of rabies virus in dog saliva samples. *Journal of Veterinary Diagnostic Investigation*, **23**(6):1197–1201. © Sage).

$$\text{Sp} = \frac{\text{True negatives}}{\text{All nonaffected}} = \frac{\text{TN}}{\text{TN} + \text{FP}} = \frac{170}{170 + 10} = \frac{170}{180} = 94.4\% \qquad (6.4)$$

This means that approximately 5 out of every 100 dogs that do not have rabies are misdiagnosed by this test as positive. What is the biological significance of this value to you?

Sensitivity refers to the accuracy of the positive results, and specificity refers to the accuracy of the negative results. Therefore, both are indicators of the ability of a test to properly classify a patient as affected or nonaffected, a measure of test performance.

For commercial kits, these measurements are calculated by the companies developing them, comparing their kit with others. As for other diagnostic tests that do not use reagents, the comparison is commonly performed by researchers that compare these diagnostic methods in controlled studies that know the true disease status of test animals, usually by controlled infection of some animals. So, most of us do not have to worry about calculating these, but we all need to be aware of the implications of using a test with low specificity or low sensitivity.

The higher the sensitivity and the specificity, the better the test is. Sensitivity and specificity over 90% are considered as high and represent useful tests. However, tests with high sensitivity and high specificity are not always available and we often have to decide between a test with higher sensitivity and lower specificity and another one with lower sensitivity and higher specificity. Which one is the best test to use? The answer is "it depends!"

- If we are more interested in making sure that there are no false-negative results (affected animals that test negative), we would require a test with the highest possible sensitivity.
- If we are trying to ensure that there are no false-positive results (nonaffected animals that test positive), we would require a test with the highest possible specificity.

Example

If we were interested in eradicating tuberculosis in the Michigan deer population, we would be interested in using a test with high sensitivity, to make sure that we have as few false-negative results as possible. We would cull all positive animals and leave only those that are test-negative to reproduce.

However, if, for example, we were testing all horses participating at an international event such as the Olympic Games for a disease that could impact world trade, we would need to make sure that we use a test with very high specificity to make sure we do not have false-positive results; it could be disastrous for economy and image of a country if a false-positive test were to be reported.

For the clinician, however, sensitivity and specificity have little meaning beyond comparing two diagnostic tests for the same condition and choosing one based on better performance. In their daily work, clinicians will test an animal and want to know how confident they can be on that result. In other words, how likely is it that an animal that has a positive test actually has the disease or that an animal that tests negative is truly not affected? This information is delivered, respectively, by the positive predictive value (PPV) and negative predictive value (NPV).

Table 6.5 Visualization of cells included in the calculation of **positive predictive value** of a diagnostic test in a 2×2 table.

		Dz	No-Dz
Diagnostic test	+	TP	FP
	−		

Positive predictive value

PPV determines the likelihood of an animal to truly be affected if it has a positive test. In other words, it looks at the proportion of test-positive animals (denominator) that are truly affected (numerator). Notice that this formula looks only at the first row of the 2×2 table (highlighted in Table 6.5)—test-positive animals.

$$PPV = \frac{\text{True positives}}{\text{All positives}} = \frac{TP}{TP + FP} = \frac{a}{a + b} \tag{6.5}$$

Some authors refer to it as the predictive value of a positive test.

Example

Following with the example of the rapid test for rabies in dog saliva (Kasempimolporn *et al.* 2011), we can calculate the PPV of this new test as (Figure 6.7)

	FAT (brain smears)		PCR (saliva)	
Strip test	+	−	+	−
+	53*	10	53	10
−	4	170	4	170
Total	57	180	57	180

FAT = fluorescent antibody test; PCR = polymerase chain reaction;
+ = positive; − = negative
* Number of saliva samples.

Figure 6.7 Identification of data needed to calculate the **positive predictive value** of a new rapid test developed for the diagnosis of rabies in dog saliva (Kasempimolporn, S., Saengseesom, W., Huadsakul, S., Boonchang, S., & Sitprija, V. (2011). Evaluation of a rapid immunochromatographic test strip for detection of rabies virus in dog saliva samples. *Journal of Veterinary Diagnostic Investigation*, **23**(6):1197–1201. © Sage).

$$PPV = \frac{\text{True positives}}{\text{All positives}} = \frac{TP}{TP + FP} = \frac{53}{53 + 10} = \frac{53}{63} = 84.1\% \tag{6.6}$$

The meaning of this number is that you can only be confident 84% of the time that a dog with a positive rapid strip test result is in fact infected with rabies. In other words, out of every 100 dogs that test positive, 16 are not infected. If you were to euthanize all positive dogs, you know that out of every 100 positive dogs, there would be 16 dogs that you would have euthanized that were not infected. Would you accept that or would you use a different test or an additional test to confirm your results? The paper never reported this value.

Table 6.6 Visualization of cells included in the calculation of **negative predictive value** of a diagnostic test in a 2×2 table.

		Dz	No-Dz
Diagnostic test	+		
	−	FN	TN

Negative predictive value

NPV indicates the likelihood of a test-negative animal to be truly nonaffected. In other words, it looks at the proportion of test-negative animals (denominator) that are truly nonaffected (numerator). Notice that this formula looks only at the second row of the 2×2 table (highlighted in Table 6.6), that is, the test-negative animals.

$$\text{NPV} = \frac{\text{True negatives}}{\text{All negatives}} = \frac{\text{TN}}{\text{TN} + \text{FN}} = \frac{d}{d+c} \tag{6.7}$$

Some authors refer to it as the predictive value of a negative test.

Example

Following with the example of the rapid test for rabies in dog saliva (Kasempimolporn *et al.* 2011), we can calculate the PPV of this new test as (Figure 6.8):

	FAT (brain smears)		PCR (saliva)	
Strip test	+	−	+	−
+	53*	10	53	10
−	4	170	4	170
Total	57	180	57	180

FAT = fluorescent antibody test; PCR = polymerase chain reaction;
+ = positive; − = negative
* Number of saliva samples.

Figure 6.8 Identification of data needed to calculate the **negative predictive value** of a new rapid test developed for the diagnosis of rabies in dog saliva (Kasempimolporn, S., Saengseesom, W., Huadsakul, S., Boonchang, S., & Sitprija, V. (2011). Evaluation of a rapid immunochromatographic test strip for detection of rabies virus in dog saliva samples. *Journal of Veterinary Diagnostic Investigation*, **23**(6):1197–1201. © Sage).

$$NPV = \frac{\text{True negatives}}{\text{All negatives}} = \frac{TN}{TN+FN} = \frac{170}{170+4} = \frac{170}{174} = 97.7\% \qquad (6.8)$$

The meaning of this number is that you can be confident almost 98% of the time that a dog with a negative rapid strip test result is in fact not infected with rabies. In other words, out of every 100 dogs that test negative, two are infected. What would be the risk of leaving these dogs in the population? Taking into account that no test is perfect, what could you do to avoid leaving these two dogs to spread the disease? The paper never reported this value.

Several factors can affect PPV and NPV, but one that is important to keep in mind as clinicians is prevalence of a disease in a population. A positive test for a rare disease is less trustworthy than a positive test for a common disease and may warrant retest or additional confirmatory tests.

Example

A positive leishmaniosis test in a dog in Alaska (low prevalence) will be less credible than a positive test in Florida (high prevalence). A positive test for listeriosis in a bison in Montana is more credible than a positive test for bovine spongiform encephalopathy.

To summarize, sensitivity and specificity refer to how well a test performs in a population of animals with known disease status by examining the columns of the 2×2 table. PPV and NPV refer to how trustworthy the results are in each tested animal by examining the rows of the 2×2 table.

The practical implication is that when looking at a single animal for which you have performed a diagnostic test, you are interested in the PPV and NPV of the test. The laboratories developing new tests need to focus on the sensitivity and specificity of the test.

As you may imagine, all four are related. The higher the sensitivity of a test, the fewer false-negative animals we will have. False-negative tests are those that the diagnostic test says are negative but are in fact affected. The more false-negative results a test has, the less its NPV is. In other words, the more false-negative results a test has, the less we can trust a negative result. A false-positive test is the one in which the diagnostic test is positive but the animal is in fact nonaffected. False-positive results are a consequence of the low specificity of a test. The more false-positive results a test returns, the less the PPV is and the less we can trust a positive result.

Sensitivity and specificity refer to how well a test performs in a population, while PPV and NPV refer to how trustworthy the results are in each tested animal.

Screening

In order to avoid possible problems related to the use of imperfect tests, clinicians may elect performing multiple tests in parallel or in series.

Parallel testing

When two or more tests are run simultaneously to diagnose the same condition, it is called **parallel testing**. In this situation, an animal is considered affected if any of the tests results are positive. This method increases sensitivity of the testing procedure because more truly positive animals will be detected. However, a problem of this testing methodology is the elevated number of false-positive animals, which accumulates with multiple tests. It is also a costly testing methodology because all animals undergo all diagnostic tests.

An example of parallel testing would be performing a CBC and a serologic test for feline leukemia at the same time and diagnosing a cat as leukemic whether positive on serology or having a high white cell blood count.

Serial testing

When testing in series, an initial test is performed and, only if this test has the result we are looking for (positive or negative), a complimentary confirmatory test is performed later. This reduces overall costs as only some animals undergo more than one test, and it also increases the specificity of the overall testing.

An example of **serial testing** would be performing a serologic test for feline leukemia only after detecting a high white blood cell count in a cat. Therefore, only cats with high blood count and positive serology would be considered to have leukemia.

Screening is a special type of serial testing where an initial diagnostic test is performed to discriminate as much as possible between affected and nonaffected individuals. Ideally, a screening test would be 100% sensitive and 100% specific.

Example

Consider we needed to test for rabies all dogs in a kennel that has been exposed to a rabid raccoon. The decision is that each dog that tests positive will be euthanized to prevent human exposure. A false positive would mean that a dog that is not infected will be euthanized, while a false negative would mean that an infected dog is not detected unless it develops clinical signs. For the sake of the dogs, it is best to choose a screening test with the highest specificity to minimize the possibility of a false positive. However, for the sake of public health, it is best to choose a screening test with the highest sensitivity to minimize the possibility of a false negative, as there may be dire consequences if a rabid dog is missed and bites a person.

However, since these types of tests practically do not exist, one will have to sacrifice either sensitivity or specificity. Which one is more important will depend on the cost and problems associated with a false-positive and a false-negative test and the ability to perform additional tests. A test with high sensitivity minimizes false negatives, while a test with high specificity minimizes false positives.

Gold standard

This section is more for philosophical consideration than direct instruction. The true status of disease has been referred to throughout the entire chapter. The question is "HOW do we determine the TRUE status?" The gold standard refers to a test that is considered to be the best in determining the true disease status. For some conditions, the gold standard may be surgical exploration, radiology, ultrasound, or ultimately necropsy. What happens with diseases that have different gradients or stages, such as leukemia in cats and Johne's disease in cattle? How do we truly know if an animal is affected so that we can evaluate how good a diagnostic test performs at different stages of disease?

Commonly, diagnostic tests are evaluated by artificially inoculating some animals with the virus or bacteria that cause a disease. In this way, all inoculated animals are considered "affected." However, we know from other diseases that not all animals exposed to an infective agent will develop the disease. Therefore, all animals considered as affected may in fact not have become affected, and this will skew the sensitivity and specificity calculations.

What would happen if a new diagnostic test is in fact better than the gold standard test until then? That is the purpose of research, anyway, to develop better diagnostic methods. But if the new methods are tested using the old methods to determine the true status of a condition, we are starting from a flawed base.

How are normal ranges for biological samples determined? There are standard procedures for this methodology now, but often the study designs are cost-prohibitive and some concessions need to be made. For example, to establish normal chemistry panel ranges, we would need to test all animals for every known disease that can alter a metabolite and make sure they are all free of those diseases before they can be sampled. As you can imagine, this would be very expensive and has not been done. Instead, animals are assumed to be "within normal limits" if they have not had any overt signs of disease. This is likely a reason why some of the normal ranges for some chemistry values are so wide.

In conclusion, always consider that the determination of the true status of a disease or condition may be flawed, and therefore the evaluation of diagnostic tests is inherently biased. Simply, be a little skeptical of test results and *do not take them as dogma*.

7   Outbreak investigations

A few times in your career you will come across an outbreak of some disease or condition where you are the main investigator. This chapter will help you navigate through the investigation in simple organized steps. One major point to consider is that often it will be impossible to determine the actual cause (pathogenic agent) of the outbreak, but it will be possible to prevent further spread by understanding how it propagates. This is in fact a very common trait of outbreaks; the transmission mechanism is identified first, and the pathogenic organism is identified later (sometimes even years later).

The quintessential example used in human literature for outbreak investigations is the publication in 1854 by Dr. John Snow "On the Mode of Communication of Cholera" (Snow 1854). He had been studying the epidemiology of cholera for many years by then and had already alluded in 1849 that the mode of transmission was through contaminated water. Through careful observation, he determined the patterns of the disease and associated it to the water supply. The causative bacteria of cholera that we all know of today, *Vibrio cholera*, was not identified until 1855.

Knowing the name of the causative agent (who) does not really help stop the present outbreak and prevent future outbreaks, but understanding the transmission mechanism (how) does. The point being not to obsess in putting a name to the cause but in stopping further disease.

> Do not focus on WHO causes disease, but on HOW disease is transmitted, so you can stop it from spreading and prevent future outbreaks.

Practical Clinical Epidemiology for the Veterinarian, First Edition. Aurora Villarroel.
© 2015 John Wiley & Sons, Inc. Published 2015 by John Wiley & Sons, Inc.
Companion website: www.wiley.com/go/villarroel/epidemiology

Definitions

First, we need to establish some basic terms used in outbreak investigations.

- **Outbreak** or **epidemic**: It defines an increase in the incidence of disease with respect to the normal baseline level in a population. Therefore, a disease incidence that can be considered as an outbreak in a city, state, country, or animal species may be considered normal in other groups of animals.
- **Endemic**: It defines the baseline incidence of disease in a population. Only emerging diseases have zero incidence, all others are present in small proportions of the population and can propagate at any point in time, given the appropriate environmental conditions.
- **Pandemic**: It is an epidemic that affects multiple regions.
- **Case**: It is an animal affected with the disease or condition under study.
- **Control**: It is an animal that is not affected with the disease or condition under study.
- **Index case**: It is the first known affected animal.

Steps in an outbreak investigation

There are five steps in an outbreak investigation that should be followed in order to ensure appropriate conclusions and can provide ourselves and others with further insight into a specific disease process. Some authors make a distinction between establishing a hypothesis, testing it, and making a conclusion, which results in a seven-step evaluation process, but for the sake of brevity all have been combined in one simple step of data analysis here.

Case definition/diagnosis verification

A case of disease needs to be clearly defined so that animals can be unequivocally classified as cases (affected) or controls (unaffected). There needs to be two clearly distinguishable groups of animals to be compared so that possible risk factors can be studied. To ensure the case definition is concise and clear, anyone should be able to classify an animal as affected or unaffected using the provided (your) case definition.

Example

Assume you are investigating an outbreak of possible salmonellosis in goats. What will be your case definition: an animal with diarrhea, an animal with bloody diarrhea, or an animal with bloody diarrhea and a temperature of $\geq 104\,F$ or will you also consider animals with other symptoms compatible with salmonellosis (i.e., respiratory)? Are you going to base your diagnosis on culture, serology, clinical signs, or a combination of two or more of these? In this latter case, all animals need to have all of the diagnostic tests performed on them to be included as a case or a control.

If you are called in to investigate an outbreak of disease diagnosed by someone else, verify the diagnosis before you start the investigation. Many times, you are called in for an outbreak investigation because there is no tentative diagnosis at that point, and people want to know what is going on. In this case, you will probably have to propose a preliminary diagnosis or simply define a case animal by the presence of a specific group of signs and a control animal by the absence of all of those signs. There may be animals that do not meet the strict definition of either cases or controls. Those animals will not be included in the analyses.

The emphasis on a written case definition may seem unnecessary, but investigating an outbreak with an unclear case definition is very frustrating and can lead to false conclusions, as well as unnecessary and unwarranted interventions.

Determine the magnitude of the problem

This will require accurate data and some calculations. It is important to collect data from all records available to determine the baseline incidence of disease in the population at hand. Sometimes, what seems like an outbreak to someone is simply a normal incidence for the confluence of specific risk factors that appear at the same time.

Example

A racetrack with a normal incidence of injuries of 1 in 100 starts is used to see one injury a week. Suddenly 1 week, they see four injuries and they think there is an increase in the rate of injuries. However, they forgot to take into account that they organized a special tournament that enrolled 420 horses, which makes the four injuries a normal-level incidence for that racetrack.

Another common example for this is the apparent increase in incidence of retained placenta in dairy farms during periods of high calving rates. The explanation is usually simple; there are more cows calving in that specific period, and therefore there is a higher (absolute) number of retained placentas, but the incidence may in fact be normal for that farm.

Note that in both cases the overestimation of incidence is caused by using "time" as a proxy for "animals at risk" for the denominator.

If you are called in to investigate a new disease, the baseline incidence should be zero. However, do not always assume that the baseline is zero; look into all available records and calculate the appropriate baseline levels. This is also a great time to teach the value of maintaining accurate records!

To calculate the magnitude of the problem, we will calculate the *affected proportion* (AP) of animals, commonly also called **attack risk**. The reason to use AP instead of attack risk (as they are the same thing) is to not induce confusion with attributable risk (AR). Remember from Chapter 6 that a risk is a proportion.

The formula to calculate the AP is

$$AP = \frac{\text{number of cases}}{\text{population at risk}} \qquad (7.1)$$

In outbreak investigations, the denominator is usually all of the population present. However, this is not always the case, and it is important to make sure that only animals at risk of the condition under study are included.

Example

You cannot include males in an investigation of abortions because males cannot abort. In the same way, nonpregnant females at the start of the outbreak should not be included in the denominator because they are not at risk of aborting.

Describe the spatial and temporal patterns of disease

To determine the *spatial pattern* of a disease, a sketch can be drawn or a blue print of the premises can be used. If the outbreak has spatial implications, a map of the area can be very useful. It is important to always make a note where the index case was found and if it had recorded movements. Then all subsequent cases should be mapped, preferably with dates.

Example

The following drawing (Figure 7.1) is a sketch of the layout of a horse farm that experienced an outbreak of equine herpes virus-1 identified as fever, abortions, and myeloencephalopathy. This sketch only represents the layout of the facility, but if we mark the areas in which affected horses were diagnosed, it becomes obvious that it was a widespread outbreak (Figure 7.2), and yet it was confined to a specific area.

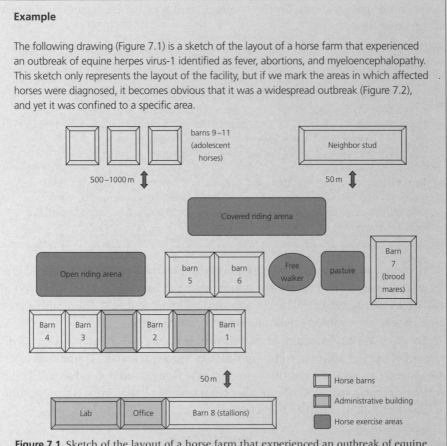

Figure 7.1 Sketch of the layout of a horse farm that experienced an outbreak of equine herpes virus-1 (Walter, J., Seeh, C., Fey, K., Bleul, U., & Osterrieder, N. (2013). Clinical observations and management of a severe equine herpesvirus type 1 outbreak with abortion and encephalomyelitis. *Acta Veterinaria Scandinavica*, **55**:19).

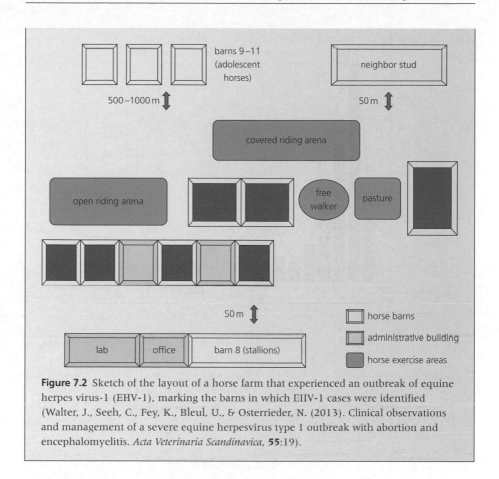

Figure 7.2 Sketch of the layout of a horse farm that experienced an outbreak of equine herpes virus-1 (EHV-1), marking the barns in which EHV-1 cases were identified (Walter, J., Seeh, C., Fey, K., Bleul, U., & Osterrieder, N. (2013). Clinical observations and management of a severe equine herpesvirus type 1 outbreak with abortion and encephalomyelitis. *Acta Veterinaria Scandinavica*, **55**:19).

To determine the *temporal pattern* of the disease, a histogram of cases per day (or cases per hour if it is something more sudden) is built to reveal the **epidemic curve**. Notice that this equates to representing the incidence of disease in the population. This will help determine if we are dealing with a potentially contagious situation or not. There are two distinctive types of epidemic curves (Figure 7.3): the point-source curve and the propagated curve.

Point-source epidemic curve

In this histogram, most of the cases will cluster at the beginning of the outbreak, with a few lagging behind. It is typically an epidemic of short duration. This is the typical epidemic curve of foodborne and waterborne outbreaks, where all animals are exposed at one point in time. Most of the animals that will show clinical signs will show them shortly after the exposure, which is why it is commonly difficult to point to one single index case. Animals that are less susceptible will take longer to show clinical signs.

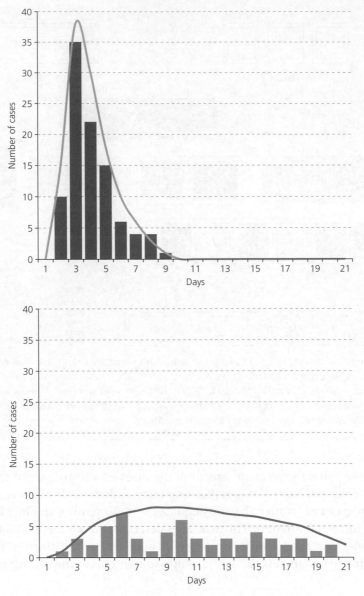

Figure 7.3 Epidemic curves: point-source (top) and propagated (bottom).

Propagated epidemic curve

In this histogram, cases appear slowly but constantly throughout time, dragging the epidemic over a certain period of time that commonly lasts days, and sometimes weeks. The index case is usually easy to determine. This is the typical epidemic curve of contagious diseases, where one animal infects a few surrounding animals, and these infect a few others over time.

Example

The following example shows the importance of the case definition along with establishing the temporal pattern in determining the type of outbreak at hand. The graph on the top (Figure 7.4) shows a histogram of the number of cows that died each day on a dairy farm that experienced an outbreak in their high-producing cows. The graph on the bottom shows data of the same outbreak with a different case definition: a down cow that did not respond to electrolyte (calcium and phosphorus) treatment and eventually died. The histogram on the top appears to be a propagated epidemic curve, while the one on the bottom is clearly a point-source epidemic curve. The outbreak was caused by a bad batch of concentrate; it was a foodborne outbreak (the point-source epidemiologic curve is the correct one).

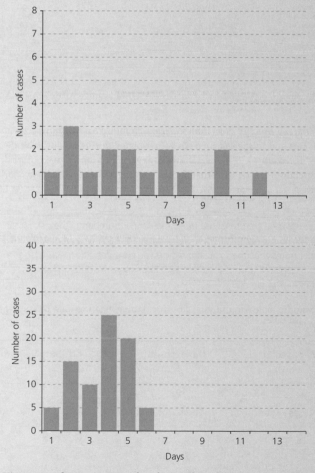

Figure 7.4 Histogram of cases in an outbreak on a dairy farm. On the graph on the top, the case definition was a dead cow, while on the graph on the bottom, the case definition was a cow that went down, did not respond to treatment, and died.

Analyze potential risk factors

To analyze potential risk factors, we will compare the AP (attack risk) between exposed and nonexposed animals for all potential exposure factors we are considering.

Example

A report was published about an outbreak of salmonellosis in military dogs in Germany (Schotte *et al.* 2007). In that report, the following table lists the potential culprits and the AP for each (Figure 7.5).

Kennel[a]	Status	No. (n)	Median age (years) (min/max)	No. of dogs (n) fed with dog feed[b]				Cases (%)[c]	Disease (%)[d]
				A	B	C	D		
"I"	Patrol duty	18	6 (2/11)	10 M	1	—		9	17 (94.4)	—
"I"	On charity	1	No data	—	—	—	1	1 (100)	—
"II"	Patrol duty	26	7 (2/11)	24 M, G	—	26 G	—	19 (73.1)	8 (30.8)
"II"	On charity	5	12 (10/14)	4 M, G	—	5 G	—	4 (80)	1 (20)
"III"	Patrol duty	14	6 (1/10)	14 M	—	—	—	7 (50)	—
"III"	On charity	3	11 (9/13)	3 M	—	—	—	2 (66.7)	—
"IV"[e]	Patrol duty	12	8 (6/10)	—	—	—	12	1 (8.3)	—
"IV"	On charity	1	12	—	—	—	1	—	—
Total		80	7 (1/14)	38	1	31	23	51 (63.8)	9 (11.3)

[a] Abbrevations indicate different kennels.
[b] A: dried mixed feed with flakes; B and C: pellet mixed feed; D: other kinds of feed (dog treats, dried mixed feed, pellet feed).
[c] Each dog from which *Salmonella* was isolated one time during outbreak met case definition.
[d] Dogs with mild, pulpy feces without fever.
[e] No sample of given feed was available for microbiological investigation.

Figure 7.5 Characteristics of dogs from a German military base from which *Salmonella* Montevideo (M) and *Salmonella* Give (G) were isolated during an outbreak (Schotte, U., Borchers, D., Wulff, C., & Geue, L. (2007). *Salmonella* Montevideo outbreak in military kennel dogs caused by contaminated commercial feed, which was only recognized through monitoring. *Veterinary Microbiology*, **119**(2–4):316–323. © Elsevier).

Notice that the data are presented using the kennel number as the risk factor, while there is no information about the number of cases for each type of diet. Therefore, we will use the kennel number as the exposure factor. The case definition was a dog from which *Salmonella* was isolated during the outbreak. To analyze the data easier, it is recommended to set up a table as in Table 7.1.

Table 7.1 Example table for analysis of outbreak investigation data to study potential exposure factors.

Exposure factors	Exposed			Nonexposed			Attributable risk	Relative risk
	Cases	Total	$AP_{exposed}$ (%)	Cases	Total	$AP_{nonexposed}$ (%)	$AP_{exposed} - AP_{nonexposed}$ (%)	$AP_{exposed} / AP_{nonexposed}$
Kennel I	18	19	95	33	61	54	41	1.75
Kennel II	23	31	74	28	49	57	17	1.30
Kennel III	9	17	53	42	63	67	−14	0.79
Kennel IV	1	13	8	50	67	75	−67	0.10

Dark gray cells are calculated cells based on data input in light gray cells.

From this table, then we need to identify the following:
- What exposure factor has the <u>largest</u> attack risk in <u>exposed</u> animals ($AP_{exposed}$)?
- What exposure factor has the <u>lowest</u> attack risk in <u>non-exposed</u> animals ($AP_{nonexposed}$)?
- What exposure factor has the <u>largest absolute number</u> of cases?
- What exposure factor has the <u>largest difference</u> in attack risk between exposed and nonexposed animals? Remember this difference in risk is called **AR** (Chapter 6): $AP_{exposed} - AP_{nonexposed}$
- What exposure factor has the <u>largest</u> **relative risk** of disease?

$$\text{Relative risk of disease in a population} = \frac{AP_{exposed}}{AP_{nonexposed}} \qquad (7.2)$$

The exposure factor that fulfills most of the aforementioned characteristics is most probably the culprit of the outbreak. The following checklist is helpful to keep track of all studied exposure factors.

Example

Following with the example aforementioned, we fill the checklist, and it will look like Table 7.2.

Table 7.2 Checklist to identify the most likely culprit among potential exposure factors in an outbreak.

Exposure factors	Largest $AP_{exposed}$	Smallest $AP_{nonexposed}$	Largest Absolute number of cases	Largest Attributable risk	Largest Relative risk
Kennel I	☑	☑	☐	☑	☑
Kennel II	☐	☐	☑	☐	☐
Kennel III	☐	☐	☐	☐	☐
Kennel IV	☐	☐	☐	☐	☐

This table shows that the most likely culprit for a case of a dog from which *Salmonella* was isolated was being housed in Kennel I.

Example

Let us review this same report now using the case definition as dogs that had pulpy feces (reported as disease). The outbreak investigation table now looks different (Table 7.3).

Table 7.3 Table for analysis of outbreak investigation data to study potential exposure factors for cases of pulpy feces in a military dog kennel in Germany.

	Exposed			Nonexposed			Attributable risk	Relative risk
Exposure factors	Cases	Total	$AP_{exposed}$ (%)	Cases	Total	$AP_{nonexposed}$ (%)	$AP_{exposed} -$ $AP_{nonexposed}$ (%)	$AP_{exposed}/$ $AP_{nonexposed}$
Kennel I	0	19	0	9	61	15	−15	0.00
Kennel II	9	31	29	0	49	0	29	∞
Kennel III	0	17	0	9	63	14	−14	0.00
Kennel IV	0	13	0	9	67	13	−13	0.00

Now we fill out the checklist (Table 7.4).

Table 7.4 Checklist to identify the most likely culprit of an outbreak of pulpy feces in a military dog kennel in Germany.

	Largest	Smallest	Largest	Largest	Largest
Exposure factors	$AP_{exposed}$	$AP_{nonexposed}$	Absolute number of cases	Attributable risk	Relative risk
Kennel I	☐	☐	☐	☐	☐
Kennel II	■	■	■	■	■
Kennel III	☐	☐	☐	☐	☐
Kennel IV	☐	☐	☐	☐	☐

Notice that when we changed the case definition, the entire table changed and now Kennel II seems the obvious culprit of the outbreak. In most outbreaks, the calculations and the checklist will not be so clear-cut, which may indicate that the evaluation could be overlooking a possible risk factor.

This is an uncommon table setup, but it is very rare to see a report of an outbreak with numbers that can be used for calculations, so this report serves the purpose as our example.

It may seem counterintuitive to use the kennel number as the exposure factor, but this is how the report was set up. There was no information about the AP of dogs that had consumed the different types of diets, which made evaluation of diets as a culprit impossible. If you read the report, you will notice that the authors actually identified Kennel II as the culprit.

Follow-up

Outbreak investigations take time. From the time when data are first available until some presumptive exposure factors are studied, it is likely that more cases will appear. It is important to include these cases in the analyses as information on them becomes available to have as much information as possible and determine the fitness of the working hypothesis. If a conclusive diagnosis is reached, it is important to divulge the information so that everyone can learn from it, especially with emerging diseases. Document all the work, write up a report, and publish it!

Glossary

Accuracy: Ability of a diagnostic test to detect the real value.

Alpha (α): Probability of making a type I error (concluding that the treatments are different when in reality they are not).

Alternative hypothesis: Assumption that there is some kind of difference between the study and the control group.

Analytical study: Study design that requires the use of statistical comparisons to make conclusions.

Association: Measurable relationship between two variables (not necessarily risk factor and outcome).

Attack risk: Proportion of animals affected in an outbreak.

Attributable risk: Measures the difference in risk of disease associated with the presence of a study variable, taking into account that there is a certain risk of disease that is due to other risk factors that are already present in the population.

Beta (β): Probability of making type II error (concluding that the treatments do not differ when in reality they do).

Bias: A tendency to a specific outcome that is not due to the true nature of the situation.

Biological significance: Importance of the results as to whether it is worth doing X to obtain Y.

Case: An animal affected with the disease or condition under study.

Case definition: A description that establishes a degree of distinctness of an animal affected by a condition.

Case report: An article that describes a new disease or condition in a single animal or a small group of animals.

Case–control study: Retrospective study design that compares risk factors between affected and nonaffected animals.

Case-fatality: Proportion of diseased animals that died due to the disease; represents the severity of a disease.

Categorical variable: Variable with subjective values.

Practical Clinical Epidemiology for the Veterinarian, First Edition. Aurora Villarroel.
© 2015 John Wiley & Sons, Inc. Published 2015 by John Wiley & Sons, Inc.
Companion website: www.wiley.com/go/villarroel/epidemiology

Causation: Measureable relationship between a risk factor and the outcome that implies the presence of the risk factor to obtain the outcome.

Clinical trial: Prospective study design in which a group of animals is exposed in a controlled manner to a potential risk factor (study group), while another group is consciously kept away from that same exposure (control group); also called **field trial**.

Cohort: A group of animals that have something in common.

Cohort study: Observational study design that follows a group of exposed and nonexposed animals over time.

Confidence interval: A range of values for a result that indicates the variability of the result if the study were performed multiple times.

Confounding: Distorting effect of a variable on the relationship of a study risk factor and the outcome.

Continuous variable: Variable with a measureable interval between values; also called **parametric variable**.

Control: An animal that is not affected with the disease or condition under study.

Control group: A group of animals that shows the baseline of normal values for the population.

Convenient sampling: Enrollment of animals influenced by external factors that determine availability.

Cross-sectional study: Study design that measures risk factors and outcomes at the same time.

Dependent variables: The outcome variables measured in a study because they are a function of other factors called **independent variables**.

Descriptive study: Study design that simply expresses common and differing characteristics between animal groups.

Detection bias: A tendency toward a specific outcome because a specific disease or condition is being detected or monitored.

Diagnostic test: A device or procedure that has the ability to differentiate a diseased individual from a nondiseased individual.

Discrimination ability: Ability of a test to differentiate between affected and nonaffected animals.

Disease-specific mortality: Number of animals that die of a specific disease within a population in a specific period of time.

Endemic: Normal or baseline incidence of disease in a population.

Epidemic: Increased incidence of disease with respect to the normal baseline level in a population; also called **outbreak**.

Epidemic curve: Graphical representation of the incidence of disease in a population.

Epidemiology: The study of diseases in a population.

Evidence-based medicine: Use of scientific evidence when making medical decisions, adapting new information and technology as it becomes available to improve outcomes.

Field trial: Prospective study design in which a group of animals is exposed in a controlled manner to a potential risk factor (study group), while another group is consciously kept away from that same exposure (control group); also called **clinical trial**.

Gold standard: A test that is considered to be the best in determining the true disease status.

Incidence: The rate at which a given population acquires or develops a certain condition.

Independent variables: Measured characteristics that are being considered as influencing factors for the studied outcomes (called therefore **dependent variables**).

Index case: The first known affected animal in an outbreak.

Information bias: A tendency towards a specific outcome because more or less information is provided on a specific disease or condition.

Interaction: Effect resulting from the action of two risk factors that are associated with the outcome.

Longitudinal study: Study design that begins with animals that are not exposed to the risk factors under investigation and before the outcome can be observed or measured; also called **prospective study**.

Morbidity: Proportion of animals affected with a specific condition in a given population.

Mortality: Number of animals that die of any cause within a population in a specific period of time.

Negative control: A control group of animals that are either not exposed to the risk factors at study (prospective studies), or have not developed the disease or condition under study (retrospective studies).

Negative predictive value: Likelihood of an animal to truly be nonaffected if it has a negative test.

Nominal variable: Variable with subjective values, commonly names.

Nonparametric variable: Variable with subjective values.

Null hypothesis: Assumption that there is no difference between the study and the control group.

Observational study: Study design that does not allow intervention, only observation of animals.

Odds ratio: Odds of disease in exposed versus nonexposed animals.

Ordinal variable: Variable with subjective values that are organized in a gradient.

Original study: An article that covers a specific question within a disease or condition, commonly aimed at showing new information.

Outbreak: Increased incidence of disease with respect to the normal baseline level in a population; also called **epidemic**.

Outcome of interest: The result of our hypothesis or inquiry.

Pandemic: An epidemic that affects multiple regions.

Parallel testing: Use of two or more diagnostic tests at the same time and considering an animal positive if it is positive to any of the tests.

Parametric variable: Variable with a measureable interval between values; also called **continuous variable**.

Placebo: A factor that is known will not have an effect on the outcome under study.

Population at risk: A group of animals that can experience the disease or condition under study.

Positive control: A group of animals that are known to be exposed to the risk factors at study (prospective studies) or are known to have developed the disease or condition under study (retrospective studies), so we can tell that the exposure is effective.

Positive predictive value: Likelihood of an animal to truly be affected if it has a positive test.

Power: Probability of correctly identifying differing treatments (concluding that the treatments are different when the treatments do in fact differ). Power is equal to $1 - \beta$.

Precision: Ability of a diagnostic test to perform consistently.

Prevalence: Proportion of animals that have a certain condition at a given time.

Preventive factor: Risk factor associated with the outcome in a manner such that exposed animals have lower risk of disease than nonexposed animals; also called **protective factor**. Typical examples are vaccines.

Proportion: Comparison of a subgroup of animals with the entire group of animals.

Prospective study: Study design that begins with animals that are not exposed to the risk factors under investigation and before the outcome can be observed or measured; also called **longitudinal study**.

Protective factor: Risk factor associated with the outcome in a manner such that exposed animals have lower risk of disease than nonexposed animals; also called **preventive factor**. Typical examples are vaccines.

P-value: Probability of an event.

Random sampling: All animals have equal probability of being selected.

Rate: Comparison of a subgroup of animals with the entire group of animals, accounting for time at risk.

Ratio: Comparison of two mutually exclusive groups of animals.

Recall bias: A tendency toward a specific outcome because a specific risk factor, disease, or condition is being remembered better than others.

Relative risk: Probability of exposed animals to develop disease versus the probability of nonexposed animals to develop disease.

Retrospective study: Study design that begins after the outcome can be observed or measured.

Review article: An in-depth summary of currently available knowledge about a disease or condition.

Risk: The probability of an event such as becoming diseased or being exposed to a factor.

Risk factor: Something that can alter the probability of an event.

Sample size: Number of animals in a group, commonly expressed as *N* or *n*.

Screening: A special type of serial testing where an initial diagnostic test is performed to discriminate as much as possible between affected and nonaffected individuals.

Selection bias: A tendency toward a specific outcome because animals with a specific disease or condition have different probability of being selected compared to control animals.

Sensitivity: Measurement of performance of a diagnostic test that establishes the ability of the test to correctly detect affected animals.

Serial testing: Use of two or more diagnostic tests, but only on a subgroup of animals, as confirmatory evidence of the result.

Specificity: Measurement of performance of a diagnostic test that establishes the ability of the test to correctly detect nonaffected animals.

Standard deviation (SD): Describes the actual variability of a measurement among animals in a group.

Standard error of the mean (SEM): Indicates the precision of measurement of the mean if we were to take different samples in a population.

Statistical significance: Probability that the results may have been due to chance alone. It is indicated by the *P*-value.

Stratified sampling: Enrollment of animals in groups and subgroups according to specific characteristics.

Study group: A group of animals that is exposed to a specific risk factor.

Subgroups: Smaller groups of animals within a study group or a control group that have certain characteristics in common. For example, males and females, or different age subgroups.

Survey: Retrospective study design that collects subjective information.

Systematic sampling: Enrollment of animals in groups at even intervals (even/odd or 1, 2, 3).

Type I error: Concluding that study groups are different when in reality they are not.

Type II error: Concluding that study groups do not differ when in reality they are different.

Variable: Any identifying characteristic that can have different values.

White paper: An article that establishes the opinion or position of the authors with respect to a disease or condition.

Formulas

Proportion: $\dfrac{A}{A+B}$ (1.1)

Ratio: $\dfrac{A}{B}$ (1.2)

Rate: $\dfrac{A}{(A+B)\text{ time}}$ (1.3)

Prevalence: $\dfrac{\text{Total no. of cases}}{\text{Population at risk}}$ (1.4)

Incidence: $\dfrac{\text{No. of new cases}}{\text{Population-time at risk}}$ (1.5)

Morbidity: $\dfrac{\text{No. of cases}}{\text{Total population}}$ (1.6)

Mortality: $\dfrac{\text{Total no. of deaths}}{\text{Total population-time at risk}}$ (1.7)

Disease-specific mortality: $\dfrac{\text{No. of deaths due to the disease}}{\text{Total population-time at risk}}$ (1.8)

Case-fatality is: $\dfrac{\text{No. of deaths due to the disease}}{\text{No. of cases}}$ (1.9)

Random number generator function in Excel: =RAND()   (4.1)

Most functional **random number** generator
function in Excel: =RANDBETWEEN(x,y)   (4.2)

Practical Clinical Epidemiology for the Veterinarian, First Edition. Aurora Villarroel.
© 2015 John Wiley & Sons, Inc. Published 2015 by John Wiley & Sons, Inc.
Companion website: www.wiley.com/go/villarroel/epidemiology

Odds ratio: $\text{OR} = \dfrac{\text{Odds of disease in exposed animals}}{\text{Odds of disease in nonexposed animals}} = \dfrac{a/c}{b/d} = \dfrac{a \cdot d}{b \cdot c}$ (5.1)

$$\text{OR} = \frac{a \cdot d}{b \cdot c} = \frac{30 \cdot 45}{20 \cdot 5} = \frac{1350}{100} = 13.5 \tag{5.2}$$

$$\text{OR} = \frac{a \cdot d}{b \cdot c} = \frac{12 \cdot 6}{132 \cdot 39} = \frac{72}{5148} = 0.014 \tag{5.3}$$

$$\frac{1}{0.014} = 71.5 \tag{5.4}$$

$$\text{OR} = \frac{a \cdot d}{b \cdot c} = \frac{39 \cdot 132}{6 \cdot 12} = \frac{5148}{72} = 71.5 \tag{5.5}$$

$$\text{OR} = \frac{a \cdot d}{b \cdot c} = \frac{41 \cdot 102}{36 \cdot 41} = \frac{4182}{1476} = 2.83 \tag{5.6}$$

Risk of exposed animals to develop disease: $\text{Risk}_{\text{exposed}} = \dfrac{a}{a+b}$ (5.7)

Risk of non-exposed animals to develop disease: $\text{Risk}_{\text{nonexposed}} = \dfrac{c}{c+d}$ (5.8)

Relative risk: $\text{RR} = \dfrac{\text{Risk that an exposed animal develops disease}}{\text{Risk that a nonexposed animal develops disease}}$ (5.9)

$$= \frac{\text{Risk}_{\text{exposed}}}{\text{Risk}_{\text{nonexposed}}} = \frac{\dfrac{a}{a+b}}{\dfrac{c}{c+d}}$$

$$\text{RR} = \frac{\text{Risk}_{\text{exposed}}}{\text{Risk}_{\text{nonexposed}}} = \frac{\dfrac{a}{a+b}}{\dfrac{c}{c+d}} = \frac{\dfrac{1}{1+26}}{\dfrac{23}{23+36}} = \frac{\dfrac{1}{27}}{\dfrac{23}{59}} = \frac{0.04}{0.39} = 0.10 \tag{5.10}$$

$$\text{RR} = \frac{\text{Risk}_{\text{exposed}}}{\text{Risk}_{\text{nonexposed}}} = \frac{\dfrac{a}{a+b}}{\dfrac{c}{c+d}} = \frac{\dfrac{23}{23+36}}{\dfrac{1}{1+26}} = \frac{\dfrac{23}{59}}{\dfrac{1}{27}} = \frac{0.39}{0.04} = 9.75 \tag{5.11}$$

Attributable risk: $\text{AR} = \text{Risk}_{\text{exposed}} - \text{Risk}_{\text{nonexposed}}$ (5.12)

Sensitivity of a diagnostic test: $\text{Se} = \dfrac{\text{True positives}}{\text{All affected}} = \dfrac{\text{TP}}{\text{TP}+\text{FN}} = \dfrac{a}{a+c}$ (6.1)

$$\text{Se} = \frac{\text{True positives}}{\text{All affected}} = \frac{\text{TP}}{\text{TP}+\text{FN}} = \frac{53}{53+4} = \frac{53}{57} = 93.0\% \tag{6.2}$$

Specificity of a diagnostic test: $Sp = \dfrac{\text{True negatives}}{\text{All nonaffected}} = \dfrac{TN}{TN + FP} = \dfrac{d}{d + b}$ (6.3)

$Sp = \dfrac{\text{True negatives}}{\text{All nonaffected}} = \dfrac{TN}{TN + FP} = \dfrac{170}{170 + 10} = \dfrac{170}{180} = 94.4\%$ (6.4)

Positive Predictive Value: $PPV = \dfrac{\text{True positives}}{\text{All positives}} = \dfrac{TP}{TP + FP} = \dfrac{a}{a + b}$ (6.5)

$PPV = \dfrac{\text{True positives}}{\text{All positives}} = \dfrac{TP}{TP + FP} = \dfrac{53}{53 + 10} = \dfrac{53}{63} = 84.1\%$ (6.6)

Negative Predictive Value: $NPV = \dfrac{\text{True negatives}}{\text{All negatives}} = \dfrac{TN}{TN + FN} = \dfrac{d}{d + c}$ (6.7)

$NPV = \dfrac{\text{True negatives}}{\text{All negatives}} = \dfrac{TN}{TN + FN} = \dfrac{170}{170 + 4} = \dfrac{170}{174} = 97.7\%$ (6.8)

Affected proportion: $AP = \dfrac{\text{number of cases}}{\text{population at risk}}$ (7.1)

Relative risk of disease in a population: $\dfrac{AP_{exposed}}{AP_{nonexposed}}$ (7.2)

Final word

This concludes the instructional part of the book. These chapters should give you an overview of how epidemiology is an essential part of the daily work of a clinician working with any species. If it has awaken your interest in epidemiology and you want to go deeper, there are multiple books that can help you expand your knowledge and become an epidemiologist. My hope is that this book will help make you a better clinician.

Practical Clinical Epidemiology for the Veterinarian, First Edition. Aurora Villarroel.
© 2015 John Wiley & Sons, Inc. Published 2015 by John Wiley & Sons, Inc.
Companion website: www.wiley.com/go/villarroel/epidemiology

References

Aguirre, G.D. 1978. Retinal degeneration associated with the feeding of dog foods to cats. *Journal of the American Veterinary Medical Association*. **172**:791–796.

Anderson, M.E., Foster, B.A., and Weese, J.S. 2013. Observational study of patient and surgeon preoperative preparation in ten companion animal clinics in Ontario, Canada. *BMC Veterinary Research*. **9**:194–199.

Anonymous. 1999. Vaccine-associated Feline Sarcoma Task Force guidelines. Diagnosis and treatment of suspected sarcomas. *Journal of the American Veterinary Medical Association*. **214**:1745.

Apley, M., Claxton, R., Davis, C., DeVeau, I., Donecker, J., Lucas, A., Neal, A., and Papich, M. 2010. Exploration of developmental approaches to companion animal antimicrobials: providing for the unmet therapeutic needs of dogs and cats. *Journal of Veterinary Pharmacology and Therapeutics*. **33**(2):196–201.

Awosanya, E.J., Nguku, P., Oyemakinde, A., and Omobowale, O. 2013. Factors associated with probable cluster of *Leptospirosis* among kennel workers in Abuja, Nigeria. *The Pan African Medical Journal*. **16**:144–149.

Barsnick, R.J., Hurcombe, S.D., Smith, P.A., Slovis, N.M., Sprayberry, K.A., Saville, W.J., and Toribio, R.E. 2011. Insulin, glucagon, and leptin in critically ill foals. *Journal of Veterinary Internal Medicine*. **25**(1):123–131.

Baumer, W., Herrling, G.M., and Feige, K. 2013. Pharmacokinetics and thrombolytic effects of the recombinant tissue-type plasminogen activator in horses. *BMC Veterinary Research*. **9**(1):158–163.

Berndtsson, L.T., Nyman, A.K., Rivera, E., and Klingeborn, B. 2011. Factors associated with the success of rabies vaccination of dogs in Sweden. *Acta Veterinaria Scandinavica*. **53**:22.

Bjornsdottir, S., Sigvaldadottir, J., Brostrom, H., Langvad, B., and Sigurdsson, A. 2006. Summer eczema in exported Icelandic horses: influence of environmental and genetic factors. *Acta Veterinaria Scandinavica*. **48**:3–6.

Boden, L. 2011. Clinical studies utilising ordinal data: pitfalls in the analysis and interpretation of clinical grading systems. *Equine Veterinary Journal*. **43**(4):383–387.

Boerman, I., Selvarajah, G.T., Nielen, M., and Kirpensteijn, J. 2012. Prognostic factors in canine appendicular osteosarcoma—a meta-analysis. *BMC Veterinary Research*. **8**:56–58.

Cazalet, E. 1977. The legal responsibilities of the veterinary surgeon arising from advances in equine cardiology and in the prescription of drugs for racehorses. *Equine Veterinary Journal*. **9**:183–185.

Cerrato, S., Brazis, P., Della Valle, M.F., Miolo, A., and Puigdemont, A. 2012. Inhibitory effect of topical adelmidrol on antigen-induced skin wheal and mast cell behavior in a canine model of allergic dermatitis. *BMC Veterinary Research*. **8**:230–238.

Clarke, D.E., Kelman, M., and Perkins, N. 2011. Effectiveness of a vegetable dental chew on periodontal disease parameters in toy breed dogs. *Journal of Veterinary Dentistry*. **28**(4):230–235.

Cook, A.K., Mankin, K.T., Saunders, A.B., Waugh, C.E., Cuddy, L.C., and Ellison, G.W. 2013. Palatal erosion and oronasal fistulation following covered nasopharyngeal stent placement in two dogs. *Irish Veterinary Journal.* **66**(1):8–13.

Cox, R., Proudman, C.J., Trawford, A.F., Burden, F., and Pinchbeck, G.L. 2007. Epidemiology of impaction colic in donkeys in the UK. *BMC Veterinary Research.* **3**:1–11.

Dean, R.S., Pfeiffer, D.U., and Adams, V.J. 2013. The incidence of feline injection site sarcomas in the United Kingdom. *BMC Veterinary Research.* **9**:17–19.

Dervisis, N.G., Dominguez, P.A., Newman, R.G., Cadile, C.D., and Kitchell, B.E. 2011. Treatment with DAV for advanced-stage hemangiosarcoma in dogs. *Journal of the American Animal Hospital Association.* **47**(3):170–178.

Ducote, J.M., Coates, J.R., Dewey, C.W., and Kennis, R.A. 1999. Suspected hypersensitivity to phenobarbital in a cat. *Journal of Feline Medicine and Surgery.* **1**:123–126.

Eddington, A.S. 1958. *The Philosophy of Physical Science: Tarner Lectures.* Cambridge: University Press.

Evans, A.S. 1978. Causation and disease: a chronological journey. The Thomas Parran lecture. *American Journal of Epidemiology.* **108**:249–258.

Fernandez-de-Mera, I.G., Gortazar, C., Vicente, J., Hofle, U., and Fierro, Y. 2003. Wild boar helminths: risks in animal translocations. *Veterinary Parasitology.* **115**(4):335–341.

Fettman, M.J., Stanton, C.A., Banks, L.L., Hamar, D.W., Johnson, D.E., Hegstad, R.L., and Johnston, S. 1997. Effects of neutering on bodyweight, metabolic rate and glucose tolerance of domestic cats. *Research in Veterinary Science.* **62**:131–136.

French, N.P., Smith, J., Edwards, G.B., and Proudman, C.J. 2002. Equine surgical colic: risk factors for postoperative complications. *Equine Veterinary Journal.* **34**(5):444–449.

Galvin, N. and Corley, K. 2010. Causes of disease and death from birth to 12 months of age in the thoroughbred horse in Ireland. *Irish Veterinary Journal.* **63**(1):37–43.

Geraghty, L., Booth, M., Rowan, N., and Fogarty, A. 2013. Investigations on the efficacy of routinely used phenotypic methods compared to genotypic approaches for the identification of staphylococcal species isolated from companion animals in Irish veterinary hospitals. *Irish Veterinary Journal.* **66**(1):7–15.

Gizzi, A.B., Oliveira, S.T., Leutenegger, C.M., Estrada, M., Kozemjakin, D.A., Stedile, R., Marcondes, M., and Biondo, A.W. 2014. Presence of infectious agents and co-infections in diarrheic dogs determined with a real-time polymerase chain reaction-based panel. *BMC Veterinary Research.* **10**(1):23.

Gonzalez Martinez, A., Santamarina Pernas, G., Dieguez Casalta, F., Suarez Rey, M.L., and De la Cruz Palomino, L.F. 2011. Risk factors associated with behavioral problems in dogs. *Journal of Veterinary Behavior: Clinical Applications and Research.* **6**(4):225–231.

Hill, A.B. 1965. The environment and disease: association or causation? *Proceedings of the Royal Society of Medicine.* **58**:295–300.

Hillyer, M.H., Taylor, F.G., Proudman, C.J., Edwards, G.B., Smith, J.E., and French, N.P. 2002. Case control study to identify risk factors for simple colonic obstruction and distension colic in horses. *Equine Veterinary Journal.* **34**(5):455–463.

Hines, D.L., Cutting, J.A., Dietrich, D.L., and Walsh, J.A. 1991. Evaluation of efficacy and safety of an inactivated virus vaccine against feline leukemia virus infection. *Journal of the American Veterinary Medical Association.* **199**:1428–1430.

Huuskonen, V., Hughes, L., and Bennett, R. 2011. Anaesthesia of three young grey seals (*Halichoerus grypus*) for fracture repair. *Irish Veterinary Journal.* **64**(1):3–64.

Jaeger, G.T., Larsen, S., and Moe, L. 2005. Stratification, blinding and placebo effect in a randomized, double blind placebo-controlled clinical trial of gold bead implantation in dogs with hip dysplasia. *Acta Veterinaria Scandinavica.* **46**(1–2):57–68.

Jaeger, G.T., Larsen, S., Soli, N., and Moe, L. 2006. Double-blind, placebo-controlled trial of the pain-relieving effects of the implantation of gold beads into dogs with hip dysplasia. *The Veterinary Record.* **158**(21):722–726.

Juvet, F., Pinilla, M., Shiel, R.E., and Mooney, C.T. 2010. Oesophageal foreign bodies in dogs: factors affecting success of endoscopic retrieval. *Irish Veterinary Journal.* **63**(3): 163–168.

Kasempimolporn, S., Saengseesom, W., Huadsakul, S., Boonchang, S., and Sitprija, V. 2011. Evaluation of a rapid immunochromatographic test strip for detection of rabies virus in dog saliva samples. *Journal of Veterinary Diagnostic Investigation.* **23**(6):1197–1201.

Kass, P.H., Barnes, W.G., Jr., Spangler, W.L., Chomel, B.B., and Culbertson, M.R. 1993. Epidemiologic evidence for a causal relation between vaccination and fibrosarcoma tumorigenesis in cats. *Journal of the American Veterinary Medical Association.* **203**:396–405.

Kilpinen, S., Spillmann, T., Syrja, P., Skrzypczak, T., Louhelainen, M., and Westermarck, E. 2011. Effect of tylosin on dogs with suspected tylosin-responsive diarrhea: a placebo-controlled, randomized, double-blinded, prospective clinical trial. *Acta Veterinaria Scandinavica.* **53**:26.

Kristiansen, V.M., Nodtvedt, A., Breen, A.M., Langeland, M., Teige, J., Goldschmidt, M., Jonasdottir, T.J., Grotmol, T., and Sorenmo, K. 2013. Effect of ovariohysterectomy at the time of tumor removal in dogs with benign mammary tumors and hyperplastic lesions: a randomized controlled clinical trial. *Journal of Veterinary Internal Medicine.* **27**(4):935–942.

Kuebelbeck, K.L., Slone, D.E., and May, K.A. 1998. Effect of omentectomy on adhesion formation in horses. *Veterinary Surgery.* **27**:132–137.

Kuhlman, G. and Rompala, R.E. 1998. The influence of dietary sources of zinc, copper and manganese on canine reproductive performance and hair mineral content. *The Journal of Nutrition.* **128**:2603S–2605S.

Linde Forsberg C. and Persson, G. 2007. A survey of dystocia in the Boxer breed. *Acta Veterinaria Scandinavica.* **49**:8.

Luescher, U.A., McKeown, D.B., and Dean, H. 1998. A cross-sectional study on compulsive behaviour (stable vices) in horses *Equine Veterinary Journal.* **30**(S27):14–18.

Malek, S., Sample, S.J., Schwartz, Z., Nemke, B., Jacobson, P.B., Cozzi, E.M., Schaefer, S.L., Bleedorn, J.A., Holzman, G., and Muir, P. 2012. Effect of analgesic therapy on clinical outcome measures in a randomized controlled trial using client-owned dogs with hip osteoarthritis. *BMC Veterinary Research.* **8**:185–188.

Malm, S., Strandberg, E., Danell, B., Audell, L., Swenson, L., and Hedhammar, A. 2007. Impact of sedation method on the diagnosis of hip and elbow dysplasia in Swedish dogs. *Preventive Veterinary Medicine.* **78**(3–4):196–209.

Mejdell, C.M., Jorgensen, G.H., Rehn, T., Fremstad, K., Keeling, L., and Boe, K.E. 2010. Reliability of an injury scoring system for horses. *Acta Veterinaria Scandinavica.* **52**:68.

Mellgren, M. and Bergvall, K. 2008. Treatment of rabbit cheyletiellosis with selamectin or ivermectin: a retrospective case study. *Acta Veterinaria Scandinavica.* **50**:1.

Morton, J.M., Dups, J.N., Anthony, N.D., and Dwyer, J.F. 2011. Epidemic curve and hazard function for occurrence of clinical equine influenza in a closed population of horses at a 3-day event in southern Queensland, Australia, 2007. *Australian Veterinary Journal.* **89**(Suppl 1):86–88.

Niedzwiedz, A., Kubiak, K., and Nicpon, J. 2013. Endoscopic findings of the stomach in pleasure horses in Poland. *Acta Veterinaria Scandinavica.* **55**:45.

Nodtvedt, A., Bergvall, K., Emanuelson, U., and Egenvall, A. 2006. Canine atopic dermatitis: validation of recorded diagnosis against practice records in 335 insured Swedish dogs. *Acta Veterinaria Scandinavica.* **48**:8–14.

Pakozdy, A., Halasz, P., and Klang, A. 2014. Epilepsy in cats: theory and practice. *Journal of Veterinary Internal Medicine.* **28**(2):255–263.

Paster, E.R., LaFond, E., Biery, D.N., Iriye, A., Gregor, T.P., Shofer, F.S., and Smith, G.K. 2005. Estimates of prevalence of hip dysplasia in golden retrievers and Rottweilers and the influence of bias on published prevalence figures. *Journal of the American Veterinary Medical Association.* **226**(3):387–392.

Pinchbeck, G.L., Clegg, P.D., Boyde, A., Barr, E.D., and Riggs, C.M. 2013. Horse-, training- and race-level risk factors for palmar/plantar osteochondral disease in the racing thoroughbred. *Equine Veterinary Journal.* **45**(5):582–586.

Saarto, E.E., Hielm-Bjorkman, A.K., Hette, K., Kuusela, E.K., Brandao, C.V., and Luna, S.P. 2010. Effect of a single acupuncture treatment on surgical wound healing in dogs: a randomized, single blinded, controlled pilot study. *Acta Veterinaria Scandinavica.* **52**:57.

Saevik, B.K., Skancke, E.M., and Trangerud, C. 2012. A longitudinal study on diarrhoea and vomiting in young dogs of four large breeds. *Acta Veterinaria Scandinavica.* **54**:8.

Sallander, M., Eliasson, J., and Hedhammar, A. 2012. Prevalence and risk factors for the development of diabetes mellitus in Swedish cats. *Acta Veterinaria Scandinavica.* **54**:61.

Samson-Himmelstjerna, G., Traversa, D., Demeler, J., Rohn, K., Milillo, P., Schurmann, S., Lia, R., Perrucci, S., di Regalbono, A.F., Beraldo, P., Barnes, H., Cobb, R., and Boeckh, A. 2009. Effects of worm control practices examined by a combined faecal egg count and questionnaire survey on horse farms in Germany, Italy and the UK. *Parasites & Vectors.* **2**(Suppl 2):S3.

Sassaki, C.Y., Colodel, M.M., Ferreira, I., Nogueira, F.S., Lucheis, S.B., Langoni, H., and Rocha, N.S. 2011. Comparison of different diagnostic tests in dogs uninfected and naturally infected with visceral leishmaniasis. *Journal of Venomous Animals and Toxins Including Tropical Diseases.* **17**:348–352.

Scarlett, J.M., Salman, M.D., New, J.G., Jr., and Kass, P.H. 1999. Reasons for relinquishment of companion animals in U.S. animal shelters: selected health and personal issues. *Journal of Applied Animal Welfare Science.* **2**:41–57.

Schneider, R., Dorn, C.R., and Taylor, D.O. 1969. Factors influencing canine mammary cancer development and postsurgical survival. *Journal of the National Cancer Institute.* **43**:1249–1261.

Schotte, U., Borchers, D., Wulff, C., and Geue, L. 2007. *Salmonella* Montevideo outbreak in military kennel dogs caused by contaminated commercial feed, which was only recognized through monitoring. *Veterinary Microbiology.* **119**(2–4):316–323.

Senior, J.M. 2013. Morbidity, mortality, and risk of general anesthesia in horses. *Veterinary Clinics of North America. Equine Practice.* **29**(1):1–18.

Silva, M.M.O., Castro, T.X., Costa, E.M., Trancoso, T.A.L., and Mendes-de-Almeida, F. 2013. Comparison of three laboratorial tests for diagnosis of canine parvovirus infection. *Arquivo Brasileiro de Medicina Veterinária e Zootecnia.* **65**(1):149–152.

Snow, J. 1854. *On the Mode of Communication of Cholera.* 2nd edn. London: Churchill J. Publications in Medicine, Surgery and Science.

Sorenmo, K.U., Shofer, F.S., and Goldschmidt, M.H. 2000. Effect of spaying and timing of spaying on survival of dogs with mammary carcinoma. *J Vet Intern Med.* **14**(3):266–270.

Spain, C.V., Scarlett, J.M., and Houpt, K.A. 2004. Long-term risks and benefits of early-age gonadectomy in dogs. *Journal of the American Veterinary Medical Association.* **224**(3):380–387.

Spika, J.S., Waterman, S.H., Hoo, G.W., St Louis, M.E., Pacer, R.E., James, S.M., Bissett, M.L., Mayer, L.W., Chiu, J.Y., and Hall, B. 1987. Chloramphenicol-resistant *Salmonella* Newport traced through hamburger to dairy farms. A major persisting source of human salmonellosis in California. *The New England Journal of Medicine.* **316**:565–570.

Thornburg, L.P. 2000. A perspective on copper and liver disease in the dog. *Journal of Veterinary Diagnostic Investigation.* **12**(2):101–110.

Tonnessen, R., Borge, K.S., Nodtvedt, A., and Indrebo, A. 2012. Canine perinatal mortality: a cohort study of 224 breeds. *Theriogenology.* **77**(9):1788–1801.

Torfs, S., Delesalle, C., Dewulf, J., Devisscher, L., and Deprez, P. 2009. Risk factors for equine postoperative ileus and effectiveness of prophylactic lidocaine. *Journal of Veterinary Internal Medicine.* **23**(3):606–611.

Toth, T., Brostrom, H., Baverud, V., Emanuelson, U., Bagge, E., Karlsson, T., and Bergvall, K. 2011. Evaluation of LHP(R) (1% hydrogen peroxide) cream versus petrolatum and untreated controls in open wounds in healthy horses: a randomized, blinded control study. *Acta Veterinaria Scandinavica*. **53**:45.

Ulleberg, T., Robben, J., Nordahl, K.M., Ulleberg, T., and Heiene, R. 2011. Plasma creatinine in dogs: intra- and inter-laboratory variation in 10 European veterinary laboratories. *Acta Veterinaria Scandinavica*. **53**:25.

Van Meter, P.E., French, J.A., Dloniak, S.M., Watts, H.E., Kolowski, J.M., and Holekamp, K.E. 2009. Fecal glucocorticoids reflect socio-ecological and anthropogenic stressors in the lives of wild spotted hyenas. *Hormones and Behavior*. **55**(2):329–337.

Vatistas, N.J., Snyder, J.R., Carlson, G., Johnson, B., Arthur, R.M., Thurmond, M., Zhou, H., and Lloyd, K.L. 1999. Cross-sectional study of gastric ulcers of the squamous mucosa in thoroughbred racehorses. *Equine Veterinary Journal. Supplement*. **29**:34–39.

Villarroel, A., McDonald, S.R., Walker, W.L., Kaiser, L., Dewell, R.D., and Dewell, G.A. 2010. A survey of reasons why veterinarians enter rural veterinary practice in the United States. *Journal of the American Veterinary Medical Association*. **236**(8):849–857.

Virgin, J.E., Goodrich, L.R., Baxter, G.M., and Rao, S. 2011. Incidence of support limb laminitis in horses treated with half limb, full limb or transfixation pin casts: a retrospective study of 113 horses (2000–2009). *Equine Veterinary Journal. Supplement*. (40):7–11.

Vos, N.J. and Ducharme, N.G. 2008. Analysis of factors influencing prognosis in foals with septic arthritis. *Irish Veterinary Journal*. **61**(2):102–106.

Wada, J.A., Sato, M., and Corcoran, M.E. 1974. Persistent seizure susceptibility and recurrent spontaneous seizures in kindled cats. *Epilepsia*. **15**:465–478.

Walter, J., Seeh, C., Fey, K., Bleul, U., and Osterrieder, N. 2013. Clinical observations and management of a severe equine herpesvirus type 1 outbreak with abortion and encephalomyelitis. *Acta Veterinaria Scandinavica*. **55**:19.

Weiss, E., Patronek, G., Slater, M., Garrison, L., and Medicus, K. 2013. Community partnering as a tool for improving live release rate in animal shelters in the United States. *Journal of Applied Animal Welfare Science*. **16**(3):221–238.

Witte, C.L., Hungerford, L.L., Papendick, R., Stalis, I.H., and Rideout, B.A. 2008. Investigation of characteristics and factors associated with avian mycobacteriosis in zoo birds. *Journal of Veterinary Diagnostic Investigation*. **20**(2):186–196.

Index

Note: Pages followed by a letter indicate a boxed note (Xn), a table (Xt) or a figure (Xf)